T0362474

Obesity

Editor

MICHAEL D. JENSEN

ENDOCRINOLOGY AND METABOLISM CLINICS OF NORTH AMERICA

www.endo.theclinics.com

Consulting Editor
ADRIANA G. IOACHIMESCU

June 2020 • Volume 49 • Number 2

ELSEVIER

1600 John F. Kennedy Boulevard • Suite 1800 • Philadelphia, Pennsylvania, 19103-2899

http://www.theclinics.com

ENDOCRINOLOGY AND METABOLISM CLINICS OF NORTH AMERICA Volume 49, Number 2
June 2020 ISSN 0889-8529, ISBN 13: 978-0-323-71306-1

Editor: Katerina Heidhausen
Developmental Editor: Nicole Congleton

Endocrinology and Metabolism Clinics of North America (ISSN 0889-8529) is published quarterly by Elsevier Inc., 360 Park Avenue South, New York, NY 10010-1710. Months of issue are March, June, September, and December. Periodicals postage paid at New York, NY and additional mailing offices. Subscription prices are USD 375.00 per year for US individuals, USD 799.00 per year for US institutions, USD 100.00 per year for US students and residents, USD 454.00 per year for Canadian individuals, USD 988.00 per year for Canadian institutions, USD 497.00 per year for international individuals, USD 988.00 per year for international institutions, USD 100.00 per year for Canadian students/residents, and USD 245.00 per year for international students/residents. To receive student/resident rate, orders must be accompanied by name of affiliated institution, date of term, and the signature of program/residency coordinator on institution letterhead. Orders will be billed at individual rate until proof of status is received. Foreign air speed delivery is included in all *Clinics* subscription prices. All prices are subject to change without notice. **POSTMASTER:** Send address changes to *Endocrinology and Metabolism Clinics of North America*, Elsevier Health Sciences Division, Subscription Customer Service, 3251 Riverport Lane, Maryland Heights, MO 63043. **Customer Service: Telephone: 1-800-654-2452** (U.S. and Canada); **1-314-447-8871** (outside U.S. and Canada). **Fax: 1-314-447-8029. E-mail: journalscustomerservice-usa@ elsevier.com (for print support); journalsonlinesupport-usa@elsevier.com (for online support)**.

Reprints. For copies of 100 or more, of articles in this publication, please contact the Commercial Rights Department, Elsevier Inc., 360 Park Avenue South, New York, NY 10010-1710; phone: +1-212-633-3874; fax: +1-212-633-3820; E-mail: reprints@elsevier.com.

Endocrinology and Metabolism Clinics of North America is covered in *MEDLINE/PubMed (Index Medicus)*, *EMBASE/Excerpta Medica*, *Current Contents/Clinical Medicine*, *Current Contents/Life Sciences*, *Science Citation Index, ISI/BIOMED, BIOSIS,* and *Chemical Abstracts*.

Contributors

CONSULTING EDITOR

ADRIANA G. IOACHIMESCU, MD, PhD, FACE
Professor of Medicine (Endocrinology) and Neurosurgery, Emory University School of Medicine, Atlanta, Georgia, USA

EDITOR

MICHAEL D. JENSEN, MD
Professor of Medicine, Tomas J. Watson, Jr, Professor in Honor of Dr. Robert L. Frye, Department of Endocrinology, Metabolism, Diabetes, and Nutrition, Mayo Clinic, Rochester, Minnesota, USA

AUTHORS

MAI CHRISTIANSEN ARLIEN-SØBORG, MD
Medical Research Laboratory, Departments of Clinical Medicine, and Endocrinology and Internal Medicine, Aarhus University Hospital, Aarhus N, Denmark

LOUIS J. ARONNE, MD, DABOM
Weill Cornell Medicine, Sanford Weill Professor of Metabolic Research, Comprehensive Weight Control Center, New York, New York, USA

AMANDA BÆK, MD
Medical Research Laboratory, Departments of Clinical Medicine, and Endocrinology and Internal Medicine, Aarhus University Hospital, Aarhus N, Denmark

ANN MOSEGAARD BAK, MD
Medical Research Laboratory, Departments of Clinical Medicine, and Endocrinology and Internal Medicine, Aarhus University Hospital, Aarhus N, Denmark

DANIEL H. BESSESEN, MD
Division of Endocrinology, Metabolism, and Diabetes, Anschutz Health and Wellness Center, University of Colorado, School of Medicine, Aurora, Colorado, USA

JEANNE M. CLARK, MD, MPH
Professor, Department of Medicine, Johns Hopkins School of Medicine, Baltimore, Maryland, USA

MARIA L. COLLAZO-CLAVELL, MD
Professor of Medicine, Mayo Clinic College of Medicine, Consultant, Division of Endocrinology, Diabetes and Nutrition, Mayo Clinic, Rochester, Minnesota, USA

AUDREY M. COLLINS, MS
Graduate Research Assistant, Healthy Lifestyle Institute, University of Pittsburgh, Pittsburgh, Pennsylvania

MARGARET L. DOW, MD
Assistant Professor of Obstetrics and Gynecology, Fellow, American College of Obstetricians and Gynecologists, Diplomate, American Board of Obesity Medicine, Mayo Clinic, Rochester, Minnesota, USA

AOIFE M. EGAN, MB, PhD
Division of Endocrinology and Diabetes, Department of Medicine, Mayo Clinic, Rochester, Minnesota, USA

KEN FUJIOKA, MD
Endocrinologist, Division of Diabetes and Endocrinology, Scripps Clinic Medical Group, San Diego, California, USA

KATHLEEN M. GAVIN, PhD
Assistant Professor, Division of Geriatric Medicine, Department of Medicine, Eastern Colorado VA Geriatric, Research, Education, and Clinical Center (GRECC), University of Colorado Anschutz Medical Campus, Aurora, Colorado, USA

KIMBERLY A. GUDZUNE, MD, MPH
Associate Professor, Department of Medicine, Johns Hopkins School of Medicine, Baltimore, Maryland, USA

MORTEN HØGILD, MD
Medical Research Laboratory, Departments of Clinical Medicine, and Endocrinology and Internal Medicine, Aarhus University Hospital, Aarhus N, Denmark

SAMANTHA R. HARRIS, MD
Endocrinologist, Division of Diabetes and Endocrinology, Scripps Clinic Medical Group, San Diego, California, USA

ASTRID HJELHOLT, MD, PhD
Medical Research Laboratory, Departments of Clinical Medicine, and Endocrinology and Internal Medicine, Aarhus University Hospital, Aarhus N, Denmark

RONALD JACKSON, MS
Graduate Research Assistant, Healthy Lifestyle Institute, University of Pittsburgh, Pittsburgh, Pennsylvania, USA

JOHN M. JAKICIC, PhD
Distinguished Professor and Director, Healthy Lifestyle Institute, University of Pittsburgh, Pittsburgh, Pennsylvania, USA

MICHAEL D. JENSEN, MD
Professor of Medicine, Tomas J. Watson, Jr, Professor in Honor of Dr. Robert L. Frye, Department of Endocrinology, Metabolism, Diabetes, and Nutrition, Mayo Clinic, Rochester, Minnesota, USA

NIELS JESSEN, MD
Steno Diabetes Center Aarhus, Department of Clinical Pharmacology, Aarhus University Hospital, Department of Biomedicine, Aarhus University, Aarhus, Denmark

REKHA B. KUMAR, MD, MS, DABOM
Division of Endocrinology, Diabetes, and Metabolism, Weill Cornell Medicine, Assistant Professor of Medicine, Comprehensive Weight Control Center, New York, New York, USA

JENS OTTO LUNDE JØRGENSEN, MD
Medical Research Laboratory, Departments of Clinical Medicine, and Endocrinology and Internal Medicine, Aarhus University Hospital, Aarhus N, Denmark

NIELS MØLLER, MD
Medical Research Laboratory, Departments of Clinical Medicine, and Endocrinology and Internal Medicine, Aarhus University Hospital, Aarhus N, Denmark

STEEN BØNLØKKE PEDERSEN, MD
Medical Research Laboratory, Departments of Clinical Medicine, and Endocrinology and Internal Medicine, Aarhus University Hospital, Aarhus N, Denmark

BJØRN RICHELSEN, MD
Medical Research Laboratory, Departments of Clinical Medicine, and Endocrinology and Internal Medicine, Aarhus University Hospital, Aarhus N, Denmark; Steno Diabetes Center Aarhus, Aarhus University Hospital, Aarhus, Denmark

RENEE J. ROGERS, PhD
Associate Professor and Director of Health and Wellness Programs, Healthy Lifestyle Institute, University of Pittsburgh, Pittsburgh, Pennsylvania, USA

MEERA SHAH, MBChB
Assistant Professor of Medicine, Mayo Clinic College of Medicine, Consultant, Division of Endocrinology, Diabetes and Nutrition, Mayo Clinic, Rochester, Minnesota, USA

LINDA M. SZYMANSKI, MD, PhD
Associate Professor of Obstetrics and Gynecology, Fellow, American College of Obstetricians and Gynecologists, Mayo Clinic, Rochester, Minnesota, USA

ADRIAN VELLA, MD
Division of Endocrinology and Diabetes, Department of Medicine, Mayo Clinic, Rochester, Minnesota, USA

Contents

Regional adipose tissue distribution differs between men and women. Differences in the accumulation of adipose tissue as well as the regulation of secretion of a number of products from adipose tissue are under the control of sex steroids, which act through a wide variety of mechanisms, both direct and indirect, to tailor metabolism to the unique needs of each sex. A fuller understanding of sex-based differences in adipose tissue function may help with tailored strategies for disease prevention and treatment and provide insights into fundamental differences in the processes that regulate nutrient homeostasis and body weight.

Although visceral fat is strongly correlated with the metabolic complications of obesity, the existing data indicate it is not the cause of these complications. Excess release of free fatty acids (FFA) from adipose tissue lipolysis can account for a sizable portion of the metabolic complications of obesity. In humans, upper-body subcutaneous adipose tissue accounts for most systemic FFA, whereas visceral fat contributes a modest portion of the excess amount to which the liver is exposed. This pattern is maintained in upper-body/visceral obesity, except that greater amounts of visceral fat expose the liver to more FFA from visceral adipose tissue lipolysis.

Growth hormone (GH) exerts IGF-I dependent protein anabolic and direct lipolytic effects. Obesity reversibly suppresses GH secretion driven by elevated FFA levels, whereas serum IGF-I levels remain normal or elevated due to elevated portal insulin levels. Fasting in lean individuals suppresses hepatic IGF-I production and increases pituitary GH release, but this pattern is less pronounced in obesity. Fasting in obesity is associated with increased sensitivity to the insulin-antagonistic effects of GH. GH

treatment in obesity induces a moderate reduction in fat mass and an increase in lean body mass but the therapeutic potential is uncertain.

Overweight and obesity in pregnancy confer a wide range of risks on
mother, fetus, and offspring throughout their lives. In addition to compounding many common pregnancy complications, including both iatrogenic preterm delivery and cesarean delivery, obesity is associated with
multiple fetal anomalies, metabolic sequelae including diabetes and
obesity, allergy and asthma, attention-deficit disorder, and likely many
other challenges for the offspring. As targeted interventions are being
developed, encouraging solid nutrition and exercise in women of childbearing age may stave off risks and mitigate obesity in the next generation.

Obesity has been identified as a multifactorial disease with several determinants, including genetic predisposition, environmental influences, dietary patterns, and physical activity factors. Iatrogenic obesity, most
commonly medication-induced weight gain, is often overlooked as a
contributing factor to a patient's obesity. This article highlights medications known to cause weight gain.

Rates of obesity counseling are low among physicians because of the lack
of time and training in this area. In recognition of this challenge, recent national guidelines encourage physicians to refer patients with obesity to
intensive, comprehensive lifestyle programs to lose weight. Some commercial weight-loss programs meet these criteria, and this article reviews
the evidence from randomized controlled trials regarding such programs'
weight-loss efficacy and safety as well as glycemic outcomes among patients with and without diabetes mellitus. A discussion of how physicians
might approach the referral process and continued management of patients participating in these programs is included.

Physical activity contributes to body weight regulation. At least 150 minutes per week of moderate-to-vigorous intensity physical activity may
be needed. When not coupled with dietary restriction, physical activity
contributes to an average weight loss of approximately 2 to 3 kg in interventions up to 6 months in duration; when added to modest dietary restriction it adds 20% additional weight loss compared with modest dietary
restriction alone. Physical activity is associated with enhanced long-term
weight loss and attenuation of weight regain and should be included within

clinical and public health approaches to prevent weight regain and to treat obesity.

There are many valid reasons why health care providers are reluctant to use pharmacotherapy for weight management: the negative track record of weight loss medications has led to numerous safety concerns, and there is lack of formal training in obesity medicine leading to a general discomfort with using these drugs. New medications have improved safety profiles, and their mechanisms are based on recent discoveries of how humans regulate weight. This, combined with a change in American health coverage, has slowly increased the utilization of obesity pharmacotherapy. This article examines the barriers and changes that are increasing the use of anti-obesity medications.

In the current setting of an obesity pandemic, there is an urgent need for minimally invasive, safe, and effective interventions for weight loss. Endoscopic bariatric procedures have been developed as an alternative to more traditional medical and surgical therapies. Multiple options are undergoing evaluation or are already available for clinical use. This review aims to describe these treatments, including their mechanisms of action, efficacy, safety and the knowledge gaps regarding their use.

As the prevalence of obesity has increased, bariatric surgery has become more common because of its proven efficacy at promoting weight loss and improving weight-related medical comorbidities. Although generally successful, bariatric surgery may also lead to complications and negatively affect health. This article highlights some common and rare complications of bariatric surgery. Specifically, it discusses the risk of nutrient deficiencies (which is influenced by surgery type) and their downstream effects, including ill-effects on bone health. Rarer complications, such as postbypass hypoglycemia and alcohol use disorder, are also discussed.

ENDOCRINOLOGY AND METABOLISM CLINICS OF NORTH AMERICA

SERIES OF RELATED INTEREST

Medical Clinics
https://www.medical.theclinics.com

VISIT THE CLINICS ONLINE!
Access your subscription at:
www.theclinics.com

Foreword
Obesity: A Closer Look

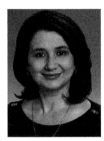

Adriana G. Ioachimescu, MD, PhD, FACE
Consulting Editor

It is my great pleasure to introduce the Obesity issue of the *Endocrinology and Metabolism Clinics of North America*. The guest editor is Dr Michael D. Jensen, Professor of Medicine, Division of Endocrinology, Mayo Clinic, Rochester, MN.

The significant progress regarding pathogenesis and management of obesity has translated into clinical practice changes with consequences for a large segment of the general population. This affects virtually all clinical practitioners, from pediatricians to family practitioners, from obstetricians to endocrinologists, and from surgeons to psychiatrists. In their daily practice, physicians and other clinical practitioners have ample opportunities to counsel patients about prevention, complications, and treatment of obesity.

Our collection of articles includes several articles on the physiology of adipose tissue, specifically, gender differences, role of visceral fat, and influence of growth hormone and insulin-like growth factor-1. These are both fascinating and impactful, with consequences on clinical preventative measures, prediction of metabolic risks, and treatment. Prevention of obesity and its complications starts before pregnancy, because obesity in pregnancy can shape the metabolism of the offspring and result in long-term problems during childhood and even adulthood.

Several classes of medications can cause weight gain, some widely prescribed, such as antidepressants or diabetes medications. These are important to identify and represent an opportunity for interdisciplinary collaboration and care coordination.

Several articles are dedicated to therapeutic interventions, including pharmacotherapy, bariatric surgery, commercial weight loss programs, and physical activity. Several forms of pharmacotherapy are available; however, only a small proportion of patients is using them. Multiple factors are contributory, including insufficient familiarity of physicians with these medications, as well as scarce insurance coverage and cost. Bariatric surgery is very effective, but patients must be closely monitored for micronutrient deficiencies, fat malabsorption, and hypoglycemia. Endoscopic treatment

Endocrinol Metab Clin N Am 49 (2020) xi–xii
https://doi.org/10.1016/j.ecl.2020.04.001
0889-8529/20/© 2020 Published by Elsevier Inc.

for obesity has become an alternative option to traditional surgical procedures with good initial weight loss, but long-term outcome studies are needed.

I hope you will find this issue of the *Endocrinology and Metabolism Clinics of North America* informative and helpful in your practice. I thank Dr Jensen for guest-editing this important collection of articles and the authors for their excellent contributions. I also would like to acknowledge the Elsevier editorial staff for their continuous support.

Adriana G. Ioachimescu, MD, PhD, FACE
Emory University School of Medicine
1365 B Clifton Road, Northeast, B6209
Atlanta, GA 30322, USA

E-mail address:
aioachi@emory.edu

Preface

Obesity 2020: From Basic Mechanisms to Clinical Pearls

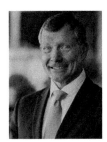

Michael D. Jensen, MD
Editor

Although there have not been a large number of therapeutic advances in the field of obesity since this topic was last addressed in *Endocrinology and Metabolism Clinics of North America*, there have been some important gains in our understanding of the regulation of adipose tissue metabolism and the nuances of the various treatment options. The first 3 articles of this issue focus on what has been learned about adipose tissue relevant to the function of various depots and the effects of endocrine factors on its function. For the remainder of this issue, we address topics of more immediate impact on patient care. One of these articles addresses what is known about the effects of obesity during pregnancy on long-term health outcomes so practitioners who see these patients understand the importance of intervening. However, judging how best to intervene is often more challenging. The first dictum of "do no harm" is addressed by reviewing what is known about iatrogenic obesity. Because many providers don't have access to high-quality nutrition/behavioral weight-loss services in their office, we address the question of which commercial weight-loss programs might be recommended. Because increased physical activity is an essential component of weight-loss maintenance, we review what is known about physical activity interventions and how to address them with patients. While there hasn't been much in the way of new pharmacotherapies for obesity, those that are available appear to be underutilized. This is in part due to the barriers often put in place for their prescribing. We hope that the article on identifying and overcoming these barriers will help providers who wish to prescribe, but struggle with the administrative burden, overcome the barriers. Finally, with the advent of more procedural approaches to obesity treatment, we felt it was important for providers to feel comfortable dealing with the inevitable patients for whom things don't go well. In summary, we hope that this issue of *Endocrinology and Metabolism Clinics of North America* provides interesting new insights into adipose tissue metabolism

Endocrinol Metab Clin N Am 49 (2020) xiii–xiv
https://doi.org/10.1016/j.ecl.2020.03.001
0889-8529/20/© 2020 Published by Elsevier Inc.

endo.theclinics.com

and a series of articles that address issues that come up on an almost daily basis in the offices of providers who deal with obesity.

Michael D. Jensen, MD
Division of Endocrinology
Endocrine Research Unit
Mayo Clinic
5-194 Joseph
Rochester, MN 55905, USA

E-mail address:
jensen@mayo.edu

Sex Differences in Adipose Tissue Function

Kathleen M. Gavin, PhD[a], Daniel H. Bessesen, MD[b],*

KEYWORDS

- Sex differences • Hormone action • Estrogen • Testosterone • Regional adiposity
- Hormone replacement therapy

KEY POINTS

- Males have less total body fat, but accumulate a disproportionate amount in the abdominal visceral compartment; women preferentially store fat in the gluteofemoral depot.
- Sex steroids play a central role in these differences by altering developmental and biochemical processes in adipocytes that are, in part, depot specific.
- Effects of sex steroids on adipocytes occur directly through hormone receptors or indirectly by modulating tissue responses to other hormones, including catecholamines and insulin.
- Emerging areas of research include sex differences in the recruitment of brown adipose tissue, disposition of bone marrow–derived adipocyte precursors, and potential independent effects of follicle-stimulating hormone.
- Although these differences have relevance for metabolic disease risk, they may inform us about differences in the priorities of fuel metabolism in men versus women.

INTRODUCTION

Women have consistently been found to have higher levels of total body adiposity than men.[1] Women preferentially deposit fat subcutaneously with greater accumulation in the gluteofemoral region. This distribution of fat may provide a buffer for fat storage during periods of positive energy balance and improve glucose metabolism, partially protecting against the development of type 2 diabetes in premenopausal women.[2] In contrast, men tend to accumulate fat in the abdominal region, in the visceral compartment, where it contributes to an increased risk for metabolic disease.[3] These differences in total lipid storage may have evolved to favor the energy needs of

a Division of Geriatric Medicine, Department of Medicine, Eastern Colorado VA Geriatric, Research, Education, and Clinical Center (GRECC), University of Colorado Anschutz Medical Campus, 12631 East 17th Avenue, Aurora, CO 80045, USA; b Division of Endocrinology, Metabolism, and Diabetes, Anschutz Health and Wellness Center, University of Colorado, School of Medicine, 12348 East Montview Boulevard, Aurora, CO 80045, USA
* Corresponding author.
E-mail address: DANIEL.BESSESEN@CUANSCHUTZ.EDU

Endocrinol Metab Clin N Am 49 (2020) 215–228
https://doi.org/10.1016/j.ecl.2020.02.008
0889-8529/20/© 2020 Elsevier Inc. All rights reserved.

endo.theclinics.com

reproduction and lactation in women and suggest fundamental differences in the handling of metabolic fuels by the two sexes. Although these sex-based differences in fat distribution could be related to genetics, the fact that these differences first appear at the onset of puberty and become less pronounced after the menopause in women or in association with declining testosterone levels in men suggest that sex steroids play a central role.[4] Studies done in human participants with sex steroid insufficiency occurring naturally or by pharmacologic suppression with our without hormone replacement support this idea. Specifically, although the increase in total fat mass seen in women with the menopausal transition is due in part to advancing age, fat redistribution away from peripheral subcutaneous depots to visceral depots seems to be specifically related to estrogen deficiency.[5] Women who receive post-menopausal hormone therapy see an age-adjusted decrease in visceral fat.[6] Men with Klinefelter syndrome not on testosterone replacement therapy have increased levels of total body fat that decreases with testosterone replacement, although hormone replacement therapy is associated with an increase in intra-abdominal fat content.[7] Studies done in transsexual individuals using gender-affirming hormone therapy show that estrogen use by male-to-female transsexuals is associated with in an increase in total body fat with relatively less fat accumulating in the visceral depot. In contrast, administration of testosterone to female-to-male transsexual individuals results in a reduction in subcutaneous fat area on MRI with a modest increase in visceral fat area.[8,9] The importance of sex steroids in adipose tissue metabolism and regional adiposity has been studied in vitro using isolated adipocytes, in studies of animals after gonadectomy with or without hormone replacement, and in studies of mice with genetic manipulations of relevant hormone signaling systems.[10] Although energy intake and energy expenditure, including energy expended in habitual physical activity, play critical roles in determining differences in total body adiposity between men and women, even these variables seem to be subject to regulation by sex steroids.[11,12] Taken together, these studies strongly support a central role of sex steroids in modifying regional adipose tissue biology, although the details of how these hormones regulate fat mass and distribution are complex.

HOW DOES ONE FAT DEPOT EXPAND RELATIVE TO OTHERS?

The mechanisms determining body fat patterning are not completely understood. **Fig. 1** outlines some of the mechanisms that could be involved in the relative expansion of one adipose tissue depot relative to another. The generation of new fat cells (adipogenesis) is necessary across the lifespan to both accommodate expansion of the adipose tissue organ owing to energy surplus, and to maintain the regular turnover of the adipocyte pool, which occurs at a rate of approximately 10% per year.[13] When responding to energy surplus, adipose tissue can expand by hypertrophy (increase in cell size) or hyperplasia (increase in cell number). The role of each of these processes in adipose tissue expansion seems to differ by depot (hypertrophy being characteristic of the abdominal depot and hyperplasia of femoral[14]) and sex (hypertrophy characteristic of adipose tissue in men and hyperplasia in women[15]), although baseline adipocyte size when weight gain occurs is also of importance.[14] Rates of apoptosis of mature adipocytes also affect the total number of adipocytes in a particular depot. Limitations of current methods for measuring adipocyte production and death in vivo in humans has impeded research in this area, although the use of the stable isotope deuterium (^2H) labeling technique has made in vivo studies possible.[16,17]

Changes in the size of an adipose tissue depot through hypertrophy also depends on the net delivery of lipid (uptake of free fatty acids [FFA], dietary fat, or very low-

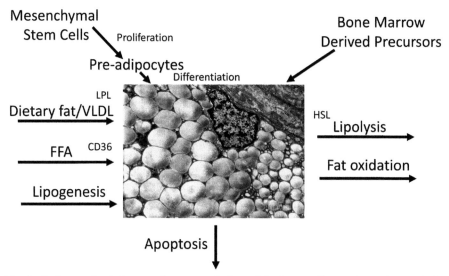

Fig. 1. Pathways the influence the accumulation of fat in an adipose tissue depot. CD36, cluster of differentiation 36; HSL, hormone-sensitive lipase.

density lipoprotein [VLDL]) and lipogenesis as balanced against the loss of lipid through lipolysis (basal or hormone stimulated) and fat oxidation. Extensive studies of the effects of sex steroids on these processes have been performed in an effort to understand the sexual dimorphism in regional adiposity.

ADIPOCYTE PRODUCTION AND TURNOVER
Sex Differences in Adipogenesis

Adipose tissue in males is characterized by more adipocyte hypertrophy, whereas females demonstrate more hyperplasia.[14,15] Tchoukalova and coworkers[14] found that women had a greater fraction of stromal vascular cells that were early differentiated adipocytes compared with men, particularly in the femoral depot.[18] They additionally found a tendency for preadipocytes from the femoral region of women to be less susceptible to apoptosis compared with subcutaneous abdominal preadipocytes. Additionally, in vivo studies in overweight and obese premenopausal women suggest that subcutaneous femoral adipose tissue has a higher capacity for adipogenesis compared with abdominal adipose tissue.[19]

Effects of Estrogen and Testosterone on Adipocyte Development

Estrogen
Human adipocyte precursors exposed to estradiol (E_2) in culture consistently demonstrate increased replication and proliferation.[20] This effect is mediated by estrogen receptors and varies with the estrogen receptor content of the adipose tissue being studied. In vivo data also support the notion that estrogen promotes adipocyte precursor proliferation in both visceral and gluteofemoral regions.[18] This finding is consistent with the overall effects of estrogen to promote adipose tissue accumulation. However, the effects are complex, with evidence also showing E_2 to be a negative regulator of adipogenesis.[21,22] The effect of E_2 seems to depend on the stage of adipocyte development considered. Estrogens seem to be more effective in promoting the

proliferation of adipocyte precursors in women compared with men, although this sex difference is not observed in vitro suggesting an important role for features of the local adipose tissue environment that have yet to be defined.[23,24]

Testosterone

Androgens seem to have a more consistent effect on adipocyte development than estrogens. In vivo and in vitro studies demonstrate decreased preadipocyte proliferation in testosterone replete conditions and testosterone incubation seems to inhibit commitment and differentiation of adipocyte precursors from men.[25–27] These results are consistent with the overall effect of testosterone to reduce adipose tissue proliferation. These effects are mediated through androgen receptors and downstream effects on IGF-1 and PPAR-γ2. Recent data suggest that the suppressive effects of testosterone on preadipocyte differentiation may depend on intermediate effects on macrophage polarization.[28]

Although androgens have been implicated as having an important role altering adipocyte development, increases in fat mass in male murine and human models of disruption of estrogen signaling and estrogen deficiency implicate estrogens in mediating some effects of androgens on fat after their aromatization to E_2.[29–31]

Bone Marrow–Derived Adipocytes

Recent evidence suggests that some adipocyte precursors come from the bone marrow in both rodents and humans.[32] These precursor cells seem to be preferentially directed toward visceral adipose tissue depots. In rodents, ovariectomy results in an increase in bone marrow–derived adipocytes in gonadal (visceral) fat as compared with control animals and this increase was prevented with estrogen replacement.[33]

Brown Adipose Tissue

Although controversial, there is increasing interest in the possible role of brown adipose tissue (BAT) in weight regulation in humans. There is evidence that sex steroids play a role in the function of BAT.[12] In both rodents and humans, females have more BAT activity than males.[34,35] Experimental studies support the notion that estrogens promote UCP1 expression, whereas testosterone decreases it.[36] In female rats, ovariectomy result in a reduction in UCP1 expression that is restored with estrogen treatment.[37]

Potential Effects of Follicle-Stimulating Hormone

As women transition through menopause, E_2 levels decrease and follicle-stimulating hormone increases. A recent study by Liu and colleagues[38] found that administration of an antibody to follicle-stimulating hormone that blocked the interaction of the hormone with its cognate receptor protected both male and female mice against high fat diet induced obesity. A similar effect was observed in mice that were genetically modified to not express the cognate receptor of follicle-stimulating hormone. In these studies, there was an increase total energy expenditure and UCP1 expression and evidence for "beiging" of white adipose tissue. It is not clear why food intake did not increase in response to increased energy expenditure, but these results raise the question as to whether some of the increase in visceral adipose tissue observed in postmenopausal women could be due in part to increases in follicle-stimulating hormone and not solely due to decreases in E_2.[39]

LIPID METABOLISM

Upper body (subcutaneous and visceral) and lower body fat depots show distinct properties in the uptake of fatty acids derived from circulating triglycerides (Tg) and FFA as well as the rates and net amounts of the release of FFA through lipolysis. Investigators have hypothesized that differences in the rate of lipid uptake and release may be responsible for the depot-specific characteristics of adipose tissue. A large number of studies over the last 30 years have examined these pathways. The results of these studies have not always been consistent nor have they supported the importance of a single pathway in explaining the observed differences in body fat distribution. Studies in this area face a number of design challenges. The processes under study are dynamic and differences in the pathways studied may be most relevant under specific circumstances (eg, during puberty, during exercise, or after overfeeding). Direct studies of visceral fat metabolism in humans are quite difficult and obtaining samples of adipose tissue from this depot in humans is rare. Data can be expressed per gram of fat, which is relevant for understanding the cellular mechanisms, or at a whole depot level, which may be more relevant for whole body metabolism. In vitro studies can provide control of experimental conditions, but may remove relevant local effectors present in vivo (e.g., local levels of estrogen or cortisol,[40,41] local sympathetic nerve activity,[42] or local adenosine levels). A number of reviews have highlighted the results of these studies.[11,23,43] What emerges is a picture of great complexity, but one where sex and sex steroids clearly play important roles.

The Uptake and Storage of Triglyceride-Derived Fatty Acids

Dietary fat is an important source of the lipid stored in adipose tissue. The rate-limiting step in the uptake of dietary fat carried in chylomicron particles (and VLDL) is thought to be lipoprotein lipase (LPL) that is made by and acts locally in adipose tissue (ATLPL). ATLPL content is increased by insulin and so, ideally, measures would be taken in both fasted and fed states. The uptake of dietary fat by adipose tissue has been examined using test meals that contain a dietary fat tracer. Tissues can then be sampled at some interval after ingestion. The specific results may depend on what time point is selected because lipid within adipose tissue is constantly turning over. Sex hormones may have a role in modulating LPL expression and activity as well as direct Tg-derived fatty acid uptake.

Sex differences in the uptake and storage of triglyceride-derived fatty acids

Meal fat studies in rats[44] and humans[45] have not shown marked sex based differences in the uptake of dietary fat by adipose tissue. Several of these studies find more dietary fat being stored in the upper body as compared with the lower body fat in both sexes.[46,47] However, when participants were overfed a high-fat meal, women stored more fat in lower body adipose tissue as compared with men.[48] Furthermore, women with lower body obesity stored more dietary fat per gram of adipose tissue in the gluteal as compared with the abdominal region, whereas men with upper body obesity stored less dietary fat in subcutaneous depots as compared with women.[49]

Effects of estrogens and testosterone on the uptake and storage of triglyceride-derived fatty acids

Estrogen Santosa and Jensen[50] found that dietary fat uptake was greater in the femoral depot in premenopausal women as compared with postmenopausal, although no group differences in ATLPL were evident. In a different study, estrogen decreased LPL and Tg accumulation in cultured adipocytes.[51] These investigators were unable to find an estrogen response element in the LPL gene and thus concluded that the effect was indirect. Yamaguchi and coworkers[52] found that ATLPL varied systematically across the estrous cycle in female rats. This variation was attributed to differences in plasma insulin concentrations during some phases of the estrous cycle and estrogen concentration in others.[52] Eckel[53] reported that ATLPL is higher in gluteofemoral fat as compared with abdominal subcutaneous fat in premenopausal women. Rebuffe-Scrive and associates[54] found that femoral ATLPL increased markedly in postmenopausal women after treatment with E$_2$ and progesterone. The results of these studies generally support the idea that estrogen favors the storage of dietary fat in lower body adipose tissue depots.

Testosterone Rebuffé-Scrive and coworkers[55] administered androgens to normal young men and found increases in abdominal ATLPL. Subsequently, this group measured the uptake of a dietary fat tracer by abdominal and femoral fat in men receiving androgens. They found supplemental androgens did not alter ATLPL or fat uptake in femoral fat, but reduced both in abdominal fat.[46] Santosa and coworkers acutely suppressed testosterone production in normal men with the gonadotropin-releasing hormone agonist Lupron. Participants were then studied before and after testosterone replacement. They found that testosterone deficiency was associated with increases in LPL in both the fasting and fed states, as well as increased uptake of dietary fat.[7] Rynders and colleagues[56] studied healthy young men once after suppression of testosterone and E$_2$ levels with a gonadotropin-releasing hormone antagonist and an aromatase inhibitor and again after testosterone add back. They found the low testosterone/estrogen condition was associated with greater lower body uptake of a dietary fat tracer. Blouin and colleagues[26] found that LPL production by adipose tissue explants declined after exposure to testosterone. Taken together, these findings are consistent with the idea that testosterone decreases the expansion of subcutaneous fat but promotes abdominal obesity by decreasing the delivery of Tg-derived fatty acid to lower body fat depots.

Lipolysis and Free Fatty Acid Release

Lipid is lost from adipose tissue through oxidation but, more important, through lipolysis resulting in the liberation of FFAs to fuel tissues and organs. Rates of lipolysis are decreased by insulin after feeding and increased by catecholamines in the fasted state and during exercise. It has long been thought that the products of visceral adipose tissue lipolysis preferentially go to the liver,[57] where they may promote VLDL synthesis and perhaps insulin resistance. It is important to note that although this finding is true in well-fed individuals, FFAs provide energy for hepatic gluconeogenesis and substrate for ketogenesis in malnourished individuals. This finding may be relevant given that the metabolic regulatory systems seem to prioritize fat storage in the visceral depot in men (why not women?).

Sex differences in lipolysis and free fatty acid release

If differences in the rate of lipolysis were the cause of differences in total body adiposity and regional fat distribution in men and women, one might think that lipolysis would be lower in women than in men and lower in regions that accumulate fat in both sexes. This is not what studies have shown. Whole body rates of lipolysis are similar in men and women and women suppress lipolysis in response to insulin to a greater extent than men.[58] In addition, women have higher rates of nonoxidative FFA disposal as compared with men.[59] Lipolysis in upper body fat is suppressed less by insulin in men than women, a result that is the opposite of what one would predict. On a whole body level, women with upper body obesity have higher rates of basal lipolysis than women with lower body obesity or lean controls, but are less responsive to the lipolytic stimulatory effects of catecholamines.[60] Lower body fat is also less responsive to stimulation by catecholamines compared with upper body fat in women.[61] Women have higher rates of lipolysis during exercise, which is associated with a greater reliance on fat oxidation as compared with men when exercising at an equivalent workload.[62] This finding seems to be due to sex-based differences in the sensitivity to $\alpha2$-adrenergic antilipolytic activation.[63]

Effects of estrogen and testosterone on lipolysis and free fatty acid release

Estrogen The effects of estrogens on lipolysis are complicated. Most in vivo studies in postmenopausal women demonstrate a suppressive effect of E_2 treatment on basal lipolysis.[64–66] This antilipolytic action of estrogen could be mediated by an increase in $\alpha2$-adrenergic receptors[67] or improved insulin-mediated suppression of lipolysis.[68] Acute E_2 treatment also seems to inhibit catecholamine stimulated lipolysis in femoral subcutaneous adipose tissue,[65] whereas chronic E_2 treatment decreases norepinephrine stimulated lipolysis in the abdominal subcutaneous adipose tissue.[69] However, studies in premenopausal women find lipolysis does not vary with alterations in E_2 over the menstrual cycle[70,71] and that chronic oral contraceptive use actually increases submaximal exercise stimulated lipolysis.[70] Local perfusion of E_2 into subcutaneous adipose tissue of premenopausal women does not alter basal lipolysis, but results in a depot-specific effect on maximally stimulated lipolysis, blunting lipolysis in the gluteal region, but potentiating it in the abdominal region.[72] Thus, the role of estrogens in regulating lipolysis varies between studies of premenopausal and postmenopausal women, adipose depots, basal or stimulated conditions, and chronic (genomic) or acute (nongenomic) exposures.

Testosterone Studies of male rodents in the late 1980s and early 1990s demonstrated a role for testosterone in the regulation of lipolysis. A study of castrated hamsters before and after testosterone supplementation found that basal and catecholamine-stimulated rates of lipolysis were decreased in the testosterone-deficient state and were restored by testosterone treatment.[73] A similar study in rats found that only stimulated, but not basal, lipolysis was altered by testosterone status.[74,75] In contrast, in studies of preadipocytes isolated from a mix of men and women of varying age and body mass index, in vitro testosterone exposure decreased both the lipolytic response to catecholamines and the expression of hormone-sensitive lipase in cells from the subcutaneous but not visceral depot.[76] In another set of studies in elderly men, testosterone supplementation did not alter systemic rates of basal lipolysis,[77] postprandial lipolysis, or responses of lipolysis to insulin.[78]

In summary, studies on the sex-based differences in lipolysis and the effects of sex steroids on the regulation of lipolysis are conflicting and do not suggest that differences in lipolysis are likely involved in, but do not play the primary role in determining adipose tissue distribution in women and men.

Sex Differences in the Uptake and Storage of Free Fatty Acid

For many years, the role that the direct uptake of FFA by adipose tissue plays in net lipid uptake was felt to be negligible. However, Jensen and colleagues[79,80] demonstrated experimentally that indeed direct uptake of FFA was a significant contributor to the overall lipid supply of adipose tissue. It is less clear whether this pathway is entirely independent of or linked to the pathway that delivers lipid from Tg-rich lipoproteins.[79] Direct uptake and storage of circulating FFA is significantly greater in the subcutaneous fat of women as compared with men.[80] Furthermore, direct uptake of FFA is greater in abdominal fat as compared with femoral fat in men, but this regional difference was not observed in women. A study of more than 80 participants confirmed the greater uptake of FFA in the subcutaneous fat of women as compared with men and showed alignment of regional FFA uptake with differences in regional adiposity with women having greater uptake of FFA in lower body fat depots and men in upper body fat.[81] FFA uptake also correlated with circulating FFA concentrations. In summary, whole body and regional direct uptake of FFA correlates with sex-based differences in whole body and regional fat accumulation.

SEX DIFFERENCES IN PRODUCTS SECRETED BY ADIPOSE TISSUE

Adipose tissue is not only a site for energy storage and liberation, but also serves an important role in the secretion of cytokines and adipokines. These secreted factors act locally and systemically to mediate a range of physiologic functions, including but not limited to insulin sensitivity, energy intake, inflammation, and blood pressure.[82] Here we discuss two important adipokines, leptin and adiponectin.

Leptin

Leptin is secreted by adipose tissue with circulating levels generally proportional to total fat mass. Because women have higher levels of adiposity than men, they also have higher circulating levels of leptin. However, many but not all[83,84] studies show that the higher level of leptin in women is maintained even after correcting for total body fat. Some of the sex-based differences in leptin concentration may be in part due to the fact that the relationship between percent body fat and leptin concentration is not linear but logarithmic.[85] Differences in leptin concentration between males and females are most pronounced during puberty when leptin seems to be important in sexual maturation.[86] There is evidence that subcutaneous adipose tissue produces more leptin per gram of fat than intra-abdominal fat.[87] Because girls and women have more subcutaneous fat relative to visceral fat than men, this factor could explain the sex-based difference. In one study, correcting for regional fat distribution indeed eliminated sex-based differences in leptin concentrations.[88] Other studies have found correlations with estrogen concentration directly. The importance of estrogen is suggested by the fact that leptin levels corrected for the increase in adiposity at puberty[89] and decrease with the menopause.[90]

Adiponectin

Adiponectin is a factor secreted by adipose tissue that is associated with improved insulin sensitivity. It also is associated with a decreased risk of cardiovascular disease. In contrast with leptin, adiponectin levels are inversely related to fat mass. Interestingly, adiponectin levels are actually higher in adult females as compared with males,[83] with an inverse correlation with visceral adipose tissue in women only.[91] The sex-based difference develops during puberty when adiponectin levels decrease dramatically in boys.[92] During this period, fat mass increases in females and decreases in males. These changes in fat mass would predict decreasing adiponectin levels in females and increasing levels in males, but the opposite is observed. In the one study that measured sex steroids, testosterone levels were inversely correlated with adiponectin levels.[93] Consistent with these data, androgen receptor-null mice have high levels of adiponectin and are insulin sensitive.[94] Low levels of adiponectin secretion from adipose tissue may in part underlie the relatively greater risk of type 2 diabetes in males.

SUMMARY

Differences in the amount and distribution of body fat between men and women are the result of a large number of complex yet coordinated adjustments to basic aspects of adipocyte biology resulting in reduced total fat but relatively more visceral fat in men and greater total fat with more subcutaneous gluteofemoral fat in women. Although we focus on the potential effects of these differences on health, the broad effects of sex steroids on adipose function suggest that lipid metabolism is fundamentally different in men as compared with women. Visceral fat, the relatively preferred site for fat accumulation in men, delivers at least some of its products of hydrolysis to the liver, supporting gluconeogenesis and ketogenesis in states of undernutrition or providing substrate for VLDL Tg synthesis in states of full nutrition. VLDL Tg is available to tissues as a source of fuel based on the hormonal regulation of LPL in that tissue by insulin and catecholamines. Conversely, subcutaneous fat releases its products of hydrolysis into the systemic circulation where these FFA are available to all tissues and their uptake is less subject to regulation by hormones. The fact that sex steroids alter so many processes in adipocyte function suggests that sex differences in lipid metabolism are important for supporting normal sex-specific functions. The implications of these differences in adipose tissue function extend to glucose and protein metabolism as well as nutrient sensing and appetite. Many questions remain, but it may be useful to try to develop a whole body model of sex differences in fuel metabolism that can be a foundation for future studies of both normal metabolism and disease risk and treatment. Understanding sex differences in adipose tissue metabolism and function may be a good place to start.

ACKNOWLEDGMENTS

The authors are supported by NIH grants R01DK114272, R01DK111622, P50 HD073063, U54 AG062319, K01 DK109053 and P30 DK048520.

DISCLOSURE

Neither author has any commercial or financial conflict of interest to report. Both authors receive funding from the NIH.

REFERENCES

1. Jensen MD. Adipose tissue and fatty acid metabolism in humans. J R Soc Med 2002;95(Suppl 42):3–7.
2. Mauvais-Jarvis F. Gender differences in glucose homeostasis and diabetes. Physiol Behav 2018;187:20–3.
3. Mathieu P, Boulanger MC, Despres JP. Ectopic visceral fat: a clinical and molecular perspective on the cardiometabolic risk. Rev Endocr Metab Disord 2014; 15(4):289–98.
4. O'Sullivan AJ. Does oestrogen allow women to store fat more efficiently? A biological advantage for fertility and gestation. Obes Rev 2009;10(2):168–77.
5. Ambikairajah A, Walsh E, Tabatabaei-Jafari H, et al. Fat mass changes during menopause: a metaanalysis. Am J Obstet Gynecol 2019;221(5):393–409.e50.
6. Papadakis GE, Hans D, Rodriguez EG, et al. Menopausal hormone therapy is associated with reduced total and visceral adiposity: the osteolaus cohort. J Clin Endocrinol Metab 2018;103(5):1948–57.

7. Host C, Bojesen A, Erlandsen M, et al. A placebo-controlled randomized study with testosterone in Klinefelter syndrome - beneficial effects on body composition. Endocr Connect 2019;8(9):1250–61.

8. Elbers JM, Asscheman H, Seidell JC, et al. Effects of sex steroid hormones on regional fat depots as assessed by magnetic resonance imaging in transsexuals. Am J Physiol 1999;276(2):E317–25.

9. Elbers JM, Giltay EJ, Teerlink T, et al. Effects of sex steroids on components of the insulin resistance syndrome in transsexual subjects. Clin Endocrinol (Oxf) 2003; 58(5):562–71.

10. Palmer BF, Clegg DJ. The sexual dimorphism of obesity. Mol Cell Endocrinol 2015;402:113–9.

11. Frank AP, de Souza Santos R, Palmer BF, et al. Determinants of body fat distribution in humans may provide insight about obesity-related health risks. J Lipid Res 2019;60(10):1710–9.

12. Gavin KM, Kohrt WM, Klemm DJ, et al. Modulation of energy expenditure by estrogens and exercise in women. Exerc Sport Sci Rev 2018;46(4):232–9.

13. Spalding KL, Arner E, Westermark PO, et al. Dynamics of fat cell turnover in humans. Nature 2008;453(7196):783–7.

14. Tchoukalova YD, Votruba SB, Tchkonia T, et al. Regional differences in cellular mechanisms of adipose tissue gain with overfeeding. Proc Natl Acad Sci U S A 2010;107(42):18226–31.

15. Tchoukalova YD, Koutsari C, Karpyak MV, et al. Subcutaneous adipocyte size and body fat distribution. Am J Clin Nutr 2008;87(1):56–63.

16. Strawford A, Antelo F, Christiansen M, et al. Adipose tissue triglyceride turnover, de novo lipogenesis, and cell proliferation in humans measured with 2H2O. Am J Physiol Endocrinol Metab 2004;286(4):E577–88.

17. Tchoukalova YD, Fitch M, Rogers PM, et al. In vivo adipogenesis in rats measured by cell kinetics in adipocytes and plastic-adherent stroma-vascular cells in response to high-fat diet and thiazolidinedione. Diabetes 2012;61(1):137–44.

18. Tchoukalova YD, Koutsari C, Votruba SB, et al. Sex- and depot-dependent differences in adipogenesis in normal-weight humans. Obesity (Silver Spring) 2010; 18(10):1875–80.

19. White UA, Fitch MD, Beyl RA, et al. Differences in in vivo cellular kinetics in abdominal and femoral subcutaneous adipose tissue in women. Diabetes 2016;65(6):1642–7.

20. Fatima LA, Campello RS, Barreto-Andrade JN, et al. Estradiol stimulates adipogenesis and Slc2a4/GLUT4 expression via ESR1-mediated activation of CEBPA. Mol Cell Endocrinol 2019;498:110447.

21. Luo F, Huang WY, Guo Y, et al. 17beta-estradiol lowers triglycerides in adipocytes via estrogen receptor alpha and it may be attenuated by inflammation. Lipids Health Dis 2017;16(1):182.

22. Newell-Fugate AE. The role of sex steroids in white adipose tissue adipocyte function. Reproduction 2017;153(4):R133–49.

23. White UA, Tchoukalova YD. Sex dimorphism and depot differences in adipose tissue function. Biochim Biophys Acta 2014;1842(3):377–92.

24. Anderson LA, McTernan PG, Barnett AH, et al. The effects of androgens and estrogens on preadipocyte proliferation in human adipose tissue: influence of gender and site. J Clin Endocrinol Metab 2001;86(10):5045–51.

25. O'Reilly MW, House PJ, Tomlinson JW. Understanding androgen action in adipose tissue. J Steroid Biochem Mol Biol 2014;143:277–84.

26. Blouin K, Nadeau M, Perreault M, et al. Effects of androgens on adipocyte differentiation and adipose tissue explant metabolism in men and women. Clin Endocrinol (Oxf) 2010;72(2):176–88.
27. Zerradi M, Dereumetz J, Boulet MM, et al. Androgens, body fat distribution and adipogenesis. Curr Obes Rep 2014;3(4):396–403.
28. Ren X, Fu X, Zhang X, et al. Testosterone regulates 3T3-L1 pre-adipocyte differentiation and epididymal fat accumulation in mice through modulating macrophage polarization. Biochem Pharmacol 2017;140:73–88.
29. Finkelstein JS, Lee H, Burnett-Bowie SA, et al. Gonadal steroids and body composition, strength, and sexual function in men. N Engl J Med 2013;369(11):1011–22.
30. Callewaert F, Venken K, Ophoff J, et al. Differential regulation of bone and body composition in male mice with combined inactivation of androgen and estrogen receptor-alpha. FASEB J 2009;23(1):232–40.
31. Jones ME, Thorburn AW, Britt KL, et al. Aromatase-deficient (ArKO) mice accumulate excess adipose tissue. J Steroid Biochem Mol Biol 2001;79(1–5):3–9.
32. Gavin KM, Gutman JA, Kohrt WM, et al. De novo generation of adipocytes from circulating progenitor cells in mouse and human adipose tissue. FASEB J 2016;30(3):1096–108.
33. Gavin KM, Sullivan TM, Kohrt WM, et al. Ovarian hormones regulate the production of adipocytes from bone marrow-derived cells. Front Endocrinol (Lausanne) 2018;9:276.
34. Ouellet V, Routhier-Labadie A, Bellemare W, et al. Outdoor temperature, age, sex, body mass index, and diabetic status determine the prevalence, mass, and glucose-uptake activity of 18F-FDG-detected BAT in humans. J Clin Endocrinol Metab 2011;96(1):192–9.
35. Rodriguez-Cuenca S, Pujol E, Justo R, et al. Sex-dependent thermogenesis, differences in mitochondrial morphology and function, and adrenergic response in brown adipose tissue. J Biol Chem 2002;277(45):42958–63.
36. Rodriguez-Cuenca S, Monjo M, Gianotti M, et al. Expression of mitochondrial biogenesis-signaling factors in brown adipocytes is influenced specifically by 17beta-estradiol, testosterone, and progesterone. Am J Physiol Endocrinol Metab 2007;292(1):E340–6.
37. Nadal-Casellas A, Proenza AM, Llado I, et al. Effects of ovariectomy and 17-beta estradiol replacement on rat brown adipose tissue mitochondrial function. Steroids 2011;76(10–11):1051–6.
38. Liu P, Ji Y, Yuen T, et al. Blocking FSH induces thermogenic adipose tissue and reduces body fat. Nature 2017;546(7656):107–12.
39. Kohrt WM, Wierman ME. Preventing fat gain by blocking follicle-stimulating hormone. N Engl J Med 2017;377(3):293–5.
40. McInnes KJ, Andersson TC, Simonyte K, et al. Association of 11beta-hydroxysteroid dehydrogenase type I expression and activity with estrogen receptor beta in adipose tissue from postmenopausal women. Menopause 2012;19(12):1347–52.
41. Dieudonne MN, Sammari A, Dos Santos E, et al. Sex steroids and leptin regulate 11beta-hydroxysteroid dehydrogenase I and P450 aromatase expressions in human preadipocytes: sex specificities. J Steroid Biochem Mol Biol 2006;99(4–5):189–96.
42. Lazzarini SJ, Wade GN. Role of sympathetic nerves in effects of estradiol on rat white adipose tissue. Am J Physiol 1991;260(1 Pt 2):R47–51.
43. Santosa S, Jensen MD. The sexual dimorphism of lipid kinetics in humans. Front Endocrinol (Lausanne) 2015;6:103.

44. Jackman MR, Kramer RE, MacLean PS, et al. Trafficking of dietary fat in obesity-prone and obesity-resistant rats. Am J Physiol Endocrinol Metab 2006;291(5): E1083–91.

45. Horton TJ, Commerford SR, Pagliassotti MJ, et al. Postprandial leg uptake of triglyceride is greater in women than in men. Am J Physiol Endocrinol Metab 2002; 283(6):E1192–202.

46. Marin P, Oden B, Bjorntorp P. Assimilation and mobilization of triglycerides in subcutaneous abdominal and femoral adipose tissue in vivo in men: effects of androgens. J Clin Endocrinol Metab 1995;80(1):239–43.

47. Votruba SB, Jensen MD. Short-term regional meal fat storage in nonobese humans is not a predictor of long-term regional fat gain. Am J Physiol Endocrinol Metab 2012;302(9):E1078–83.

48. Votruba SB, Jensen MD. Sex-specific differences in leg fat uptake are revealed with a high-fat meal. Am J Physiol Endocrinol Metab 2006;291(5):E1115–23.

49. Santosa S, Hensrud DD, Votruba SB, et al. The influence of sex and obesity phenotype on meal fatty acid metabolism before and after weight loss. Am J Clin Nutr 2008;88(4):1134–41.

50. Santosa S, Jensen MD. Adipocyte fatty acid storage factors enhance subcutaneous fat storage in postmenopausal women. Diabetes 2013;62(3):775–82.

51. Homma H, Kurachi H, Nishio Y, et al. Estrogen suppresses transcription of lipoprotein lipase gene. Existence of a unique estrogen response element on the lipoprotein lipase promoter. J Biol Chem 2000;275(15):11404–11.

52. Yamaguchi M, Katoh S, Morimoto C, et al. The hormonal responses of lipoprotein lipase activity and lipolysis in adipose tissue differ depending on the stage of the estrous cycle in female rats. Int J Obes Relat Metab Disord 2002;26(5):610–7.

53. Eckel RH. Lipoprotein lipase. A multifunctional enzyme relevant to common metabolic diseases. N Engl J Med 1989;320(16):1060–8.

54. Rebuffe-Scrive M, Lonnroth P, Marin P, et al. Regional adipose tissue metabolism in men and postmenopausal women. Int J Obes 1987;11(4):347–55.

55. Rebuffe-Scrive M, Marin P, Bjorntorp P. Effect of testosterone on abdominal adipose tissue in men. Int J Obes 1991;15(11):791–5.

56. Rynders CA, Schmidt SL, Bergouignan A, et al. Effects of short-term sex steroid suppression on dietary fat storage patterns in healthy males. Physiol Rep 2018; 6(2). https://doi.org/10.14814/phy2.13533.

57. Nielsen S, Guo Z, Johnson CM, et al. Splanchnic lipolysis in human obesity. J Clin Invest 2004;113(11):1582–8.

58. Jensen MD. Gender differences in regional fatty acid metabolism before and after meal ingestion. J Clin Invest 1995;96(5):2297–303.

59. Koutsari C, Basu R, Rizza RA, et al. Nonoxidative free fatty acid disposal is greater in young women than men. J Clin Endocrinol Metab 2011;96(2):541–7.

60. Jensen MD, Haymond MW, Rizza RA, et al. Influence of body fat distribution on free fatty acid metabolism in obesity. J Clin Invest 1989;83(4):1168–73.

61. Guo Z, Johnson CM, Jensen MD. Regional lipolytic responses to isoproterenol in women. Am J Physiol 1997;273(1 Pt 1):E108–12.

62. Tarnopolsky MA. Sex differences in exercise metabolism and the role of 17-beta estradiol. Med Sci Sports Exerc 2008;40(4):648–54.

63. Schmidt SL, Bessesen DH, Stotz S, et al. Adrenergic control of lipolysis in women compared with men. J Appl Physiol (1985) 2014;117(9):1008–19.

64. Jensen MD, Martin ML, Cryer PE, et al. Effects of estrogen on free fatty acid metabolism in humans. Am J Physiol 1994;266(6 Pt 1):E914–20.

65. Gormsen LC, Host C, Hjerrild BE, et al. Estradiol acutely inhibits whole body lipid oxidation and attenuates lipolysis in subcutaneous adipose tissue: a randomized, placebo-controlled study in postmenopausal women. Eur J Endocrinol 2012; 167(4):543–51.

66. Van Pelt RE, Gozansky WS, Hickner RC, et al. Acute modulation of adipose tissue lipolysis by intravenous estrogens. Obesity (Silver Spring) 2006;14(12):2163–72.

67. Pedersen SB, Kristensen K, Hermann PA, et al. Estrogen controls lipolysis by up-regulating alpha2A-adrenergic receptors directly in human adipose tissue through the estrogen receptor alpha. Implications for the female fat distribution. J Clin Endocrinol Metab 2004;89(4):1869–78.

68. Pereira RI, Casey BA, Swibas TA, et al. Timing of estradiol treatment after meno-pause may determine benefit or harm to insulin action. J Clin Endocrinol Metab 2015;100(12):4456–62.

69. Lindberg UB, Crona N, Silfverstolpe G, et al. Regional adipose tissue metabolism in postmenopausal women after treatment with exogenous sex steroids. Horm Metab Res 1990;22(6):345–51.

70. Casazza GA, Jacobs KA, Suh SH, et al. Menstrual cycle phase and oral contra-ceptive effects on triglyceride mobilization during exercise. J Appl Physiol (1985) 2004;97(1):302–9.

71. Horton TJ, Miller EK, Bourret K. No effect of menstrual cycle phase on glycerol or palmitate kinetics during 90 min of moderate exercise. J Appl Physiol (1985) 2006;100(3):917–25.

72. Gavin KM, Cooper EE, Raymer DK, et al. Estradiol effects on subcutaneous ad-ipose tissue lipolysis in premenopausal women are adipose tissue depot specific and treatment dependent. Am J Physiol Endocrinol Metab 2013;304(11): E1167–74.

73. Pecquery R, Leneveu MC, Giudicelli Y. Influence of androgenic status on the alpha 2/beta-adrenergic control of lipolysis in white fat cells: predominant alpha 2-antilipolytic response in testosterone-treated-castrated hamsters. Endocri-nology 1988;122(6):2590–6.

74. Xu X, De Pergola G, Bjorntorp P. The effects of androgens on the regulation of lipolysis in adipose precursor cells. Endocrinology 1990;126(2):1229–34.

75. Xu XF, De Pergola G, Bjorntorp P. Testosterone increases lipolysis and the num-ber of beta-adrenoceptors in male rat adipocytes. Endocrinology 1991;128(1): 379–82.

76. Dicker A, Ryden M, Naslund E, et al. Effect of testosterone on lipolysis in human pre-adipocytes from different fat depots. Diabetologia 2004;47(3):420–8.

77. Koutsari C, Ali AH, Nair KS, et al. Fatty acid metabolism in the elderly: effects of dehydroepiandrosterone and testosterone replacement in hormonally deficient men and women. J Clin Endocrinol Metab 2009;94(9):3414–23.

78. Espinosa De Ycaza AE, Rizza RA, Nair KS, et al. Effect of dehydroepiandroster-one and testosterone supplementation on systemic lipolysis. J Clin Endocrinol Metab 2016;101(4):1719–28.

79. Sondergaard E, Gormsen LC, Nellemann B, et al. Body composition determines direct FFA storage pattern in overweight women. Am J Physiol Endocrinol Metab 2012;302(12):E1599–604.

80. Shadid S, Koutsari C, Jensen MD. Direct free fatty acid uptake into human adipo-cytes in vivo: relation to body fat distribution. Diabetes 2007;56(5):1369–75.

81. Koutsari C, Ali AH, Mundi MS, et al. Storage of circulating free fatty acid in adi-pose tissue of postabsorptive humans: quantitative measures and implications for body fat distribution. Diabetes 2011;60(8):2032–40.

82. Fasshauer M, Bluher M. Adipokines in health and disease. Trends Pharmacol Sci 2015;36(7):461–70.

83. Christen T, Trompet S, Noordam R, et al. Sex differences in body fat distribution are related to sex differences in serum leptin and adiponectin. Peptides 2018; 107:25–31.

84. Hunma S, Ramuth H, Miles-Chan JL, et al. Do gender and ethnic differences in fasting leptin in Indians and Creoles of Mauritius persist beyond differences in adiposity? Int J Obes (Lond) 2018;42(2):280–3.

85. Jensen MD, Hensrud D, O'Brien PC, et al. Collection and interpretation of plasma leptin concentration data in humans. Obes Res 1999;7(3):241–5.

86. Horlick MB, Rosenbaum M, Nicolson M, et al. Effect of puberty on the relationship between circulating leptin and body composition. J Clin Endocrinol Metab 2000; 85(7):2509–18.

87. Montague CT, Prins JB, Sanders L, et al. Depot- and sex-specific differences in human leptin mRNA expression: implications for the control of regional fat distribution. Diabetes 1997;46(3):342–7.

88. Nagy TR, Gower BA, Trowbridge CA, et al. Effects of gender, ethnicity, body composition, and fat distribution on serum leptin concentrations in children. J Clin Endocrinol Metab 1997;82(7):2148–52.

89. Ahmed ML, Ong KK, Morrell DJ, et al. Longitudinal study of leptin concentrations during puberty: sex differences and relationship to changes in body composition. J Clin Endocrinol Metab 1999;84(3):899–905.

90. Isidori AM, Strollo F, More M, et al. Leptin and aging: correlation with endocrine changes in male and female healthy adult populations of different body weights. J Clin Endocrinol Metab 2000;85(5):1954–62.

91. Bidulescu A, Liu J, Hickson DA, et al. Gender differences in the association of visceral and subcutaneous adiposity with adiponectin in African Americans: the Jackson Heart Study. BMC Cardiovasc Disord 2013;13:9.

92. Ohman-Hanson RA, Cree-Green M, Kelsey MM, et al. Ethnic and sex differences in adiponectin: from childhood to adulthood. J Clin Endocrinol Metab 2016; 101(12):4808–15.

93. Bottner A, Kratzsch J, Muller G, et al. Gender differences of adiponectin levels develop during the progression of puberty and are related to serum androgen levels. J Clin Endocrinol Metab 2004;89(8):4053–61.

94. Fan W, Yanase T, Nomura M, et al. Androgen receptor null male mice develop late-onset obesity caused by decreased energy expenditure and lipolytic activity but show normal insulin sensitivity with high adiponectin secretion. Diabetes 2005;54(4):1000–8.

Visceral Fat: Culprit or Canary?

Michael D. Jensen, MD

KEYWORDS

- Adipose tissue • Free fatty acids • Insulin resistance • Adipogenesis

KEY POINTS

- Excess free fatty acid (FFA) release from adipose tissue can cause tissue dysfunction/insulin resistance.
- Most systemic FFA comes from upper-body subcutaneous fat.
- Visceral fat FFA release may disproportionately affect the liver.
- Visceral fat gain is associated with dysfunctional subcutaneous adipose function, not the cause of it.
- Adipocyte hypertrophy appears to be the common denominator for dysfunctional adipose tissue.

INTRODUCTION

Upper-body/visceral obesity increases the risk for dyslipidemia,[1] hypertension,[2,3] and type 2 diabetes,[4,5] whereas relatively greater amounts of lower-body fat are independently associated with a lesser risk of insulin resistance and associated metabolic abnormalities.[6] Many,[7–9] but not all[10] reports indicate that visceral fat is more strongly associated with abnormal metabolic profiles than upper-body subcutaneous fat. The obvious hypothesis is that visceral fat is doing something that directly contributes to insulin resistance. Because the primary functions of adipose tissue are the regulated storage/release of fatty acids and secretion of adipokines, many presume that abnormalities of one of these functions, perhaps combined with the unique anatomy of visceral fat, is the culprit.

ANATOMY OF VISCERAL AND SUBCUTANEOUS FAT: STRUCTURE AND FUNCTIONS

Each of the major fat depots has unique characteristics. Upper-body subcutaneous fat includes superficial and deep truncal depots,[11,12] upper-extremity fat, and, in women, breast adipose tissue. Upper-body subcutaneous fat is usually the largest depot. For purposes of simplicity, lower-body subcutaneous fat can be summed to include gluteal, femoral, and calf adipose tissue, although there is evidence that gluteal fat and thigh fat are somewhat different.[13] The lower-body fat depot is

Department of Endocrinology, Metabolism, Diabetes, & Nutrition, Mayo Clinic, 200 First Street Southwest, Room 5-194 Joseph, Rochester, MN 55905, USA
E-mail address: jensen@mayo.edu

Endocrinol Metab Clin N Am 49 (2020) 229–237
https://doi.org/10.1016/j.ecl.2020.02.002
0889-8529/20/© 2020 Elsevier Inc. All rights reserved.

endo.theclinics.com

commonly demarcated as all adipose tissue caudal to the inguinal ligament anteriorly and the ileac crest posteriorly. There is also adipose tissue in between the major muscle groups (so-called marbling).[14] Intraabdominal fat includes omental and mesenteric (visceral) depots, both of which drain into the portal vein, as well as perinephric fat, which drains into the systemic circulation. Subcutaneous and visceral fat depots have different supporting structural features, including the directionality of the septa that carry the vascular and nerve supplies. Like almost all other tissues, adipose tissue has its own arterial supply system that delivers nutrients and its own venous system that drains into the systemic venous circulation, or in the case of mesenteric and omental fat, into the portal circulation. The adipose tissue "marbling" in muscle, pancreas, and pericardial fat has this same vascular arrangement. The only exceptions are adipocytes in the bone marrow, breast, and the epicardium; these adipocytes abut nonadipose tissue cells and thus can directly affect the function of adjacent cells independent of the circulation. The major adipose depots described above also differ in terms of the average size of the adipocytes,[13] the responsiveness of the adipocytes to prolipolytic and antilipolytic hormones,[15–17] the propensity of the adipocytes to take up and store fatty acids,[18–20] as well as immune cell infiltration.[21]

The utilitarian rationale for defining human body fat compartments into lower-body fat, upper-body subcutaneous fat, and intraabdominal/visceral fat rests on the fact that the compartments can be measured using only dual-energy x-ray absorptiometry and a single-slice computed tomographic or MRI scan of the abdomen.[22,23] For those with the time and technical expertise, it is possible to use MRI to define the numerous subdepots of adipose tissue.[12]

Although the adipocytes within each depot carry out similar functions in general, storage of fatty acids as triglycerides, release of free fatty acids (FFA) via lipolysis, and secretion of adipokines, there is considerable heterogeneity in the propensity of these depots to respond to various stimuli that determine the overall effect of body fat on metabolic functions. In addition to adipocytes, adipose tissue comprises the vascular supply cells (endothelial cells and so forth), preadipocytes, and immune cells, most notably, but not exclusively, macrophages. An excess macrophage burden in adipose tissue is thought to represent a low-grade, sterile inflammatory response that might be responsible for phenomena ranging from local adipocyte dysfunction to systemic inflammation. Despite the many interesting animal models that implicate inflammation in a variety of metabolic problems, there are insufficient data to define how adipose tissue macrophages in humans impact health and disease. Visceral fat depots have a greater number of macrophages than subcutaneous fat,[24] even in normal-weight adults, which may reflect the importance of this depot with regards to protecting humans from uncontrolled spread of bacteria that gain access to the peritoneal cavity.

In addition to the proposed inflammatory properties of macrophages, it has been shown that senescent preadipocytes can induce inflammation.[25] Senescence occurs when cells are no longer able to replicate and are unable to undergo terminal differentiation (to mature adipocytes in the case of preadipocytes). Senescent preadipocytes secrete proinflammatory proteins and chemoattractant molecules that can cause the accumulation of macrophages.

ASSOCIATIONS BETWEEN VISCERAL FAT AND METABOLIC HEALTH

As noted above, visceral fat is a stronger predictor of insulin resistance–related illnesses than is body mass index. Increased visceral fat is associated with glucose intolerance,[26] and insulin sensitivity correlates with visceral fat mass in normal adults[27,28] and in people with type 2 diabetes.[29,30] There is also a strong correlation between visceral fat and circulating very-low-density lipoprotein (VLDL) triglyceride concentrations,[26] which may relate to greater delivery of FFA to the liver from visceral adipose tissue lipolysis.[31]

In vitro studies have shown that omental adipocytes have greater lipolytic potential than fat cells from subcutaneous adipose tissue.[32] Thus, the argument is that visceral fat adipocytes in humans with visceral obesity, being more lipolytically active, will deliver large amounts of FFA directly into the portal vein, exposing both the liver and, via the hepatic vein, peripheral tissues, to higher FFA concentrations. It was previously thought that much of the excess systemic FFA seen in upper-body obesity originated from accelerated lipolysis in visceral fat. However, the only tissue that appears disproportionately impacted by visceral adipose tissue lipolysis is the liver; the proportion of FFA to which the liver is exposed is correlated with visceral fat,[33] whereas most of the systemic FFA (those that are seen by muscle and so forth) come from subcutaneous fat. The author found that the degree of failure of insulin to suppress adipose tissue lipolysis from upper-body subcutaneous fat is correlated with visceral fat,[34] which might suggest that visceral fat has some direct effect on the function of subcutaneous fat.

WHAT IS KNOWN ABOUT VISCERAL ADIPOSE TISSUE: FAT STORAGE, LIPOLYSIS, AND ADIPOKINES?

Studies of visceral adipocytes using in vitro techniques are numerous. However, extrapolating from in vitro studies to in vivo physiology is challenging. The data generated from such studies often examine parameters such as maximum rates of lipolysis (which seldom occurs in vivo), messenger RNA content, protein content, or enzyme activities as surrogates for in vivo function. In addition, data are frequently expressed relative to cell number with little consideration for how cell number/size relates to depot size and therefore physiologic impacts. Few investigators have measured the concentrations of FFA in the portal vein in vivo, in humans,[35] presumably the site that is most influenced by lipolysis from visceral fat depots. Unfortunately, this seminal paper did not provide arterial FFA concentrations that would allow more insights into FFA release from visceral fat. There have been measurements of cytokine release into the portal vein from visceral fat[36] and into the venous effluent of abdominal subcutaneous[37] fat. Net release of interleukin-6 (IL-6) has been detected from both depots, and the concentration of IL-6 in the portal vein is associated with inflammation as measured by C-reactive protein (CRP),[36] suggesting that the liver is impacted by release of cytokines, in addition to FFA, from visceral fat.

More has been learned about the fatty acid storage characteristics of visceral fat and how they differ from subcutaneous fat depots, which is surprisingly helpful when thinking about lipolysis rates. Studies of how dietary fat,[18,20,38] VLDL-triglyceride fatty acids,[39] and direct FFA storage[40,41] in visceral adipose tissue have been conducted. A counterintuitive finding from studies of fatty acid storage in visceral fat is that humans with more visceral fat do not store more fatty acids. In fact, some studies found that the greatest efficiency of storage is in those with the smallest visceral fat depots.[20,40] The reduced storage of fatty acids as a function of visceral fat mass mirrors the downregulation of proteins and enzymes responsible for fatty acid transport into the cells and conversion of nonesterified fatty acids into triglycerides.[40] This finding is in contrast to the tendency of fat storage (and adipocyte fatty acid storage factors) to remain stable (abdominal fat) or actually increase (femoral fat) as a function of depot size.[20]

In order for visceral fat to be able to release FFA in amounts needed to create excess systemic FFA, visceral fat would need to preferentially take up and store fatty acids as a prerequisite to expand. Instead, the available data indicate that visceral fat downregulates the fat storage processes as it expands. How can visceral fat to continue to increase in mass despite downregulation of fatty acid storage pathways? There must be an even greater downregulation of lipolysis pathways and/or visceral fat is exposed to conditions that drive fatty acids into this depot. Because visceral obesity is associated with failure to normally suppress lipolysis after meals[42,43] as well as higher postprandial chylomicron concentrations,[43] it is possible that the higher FFA and chylomicron-triglyceride concentrations drive fatty acids into ectopic depots, including visceral fat. The dysfunction of subcutaneous adipose tissue in terms of excess FFA release may drive visceral adipose fatty acid storage via the direct storage pathway; greater uptake of FFA in the splanchnic bed under postprandial conditions has been reported in visceral obesity.[43]

FREE FATTY ACID EFFECTS ON TISSUE FUNCTION

Although the delivery of FFA from adipose tissue into the circulation to provide fuel for lean tissue is vital for normal tissue function, there is ample evidence that excess FFA induces insulin resistance in humans[44–46] by interfering with insulin signaling.[47] Furthermore, short-term suppression of lipolysis with Acipimox in obese humans improves the suppression of hepatic glucose production[48] and stimulates muscle glucose uptake.[49] In animal models, it is possible to manipulate lipolysis using nonpharmacologic approaches; these studies show similar benefits. Hormone-sensitive lipase haploinsufficient obese mice have lower adipose tissue lipolysis rates and much better insulin sensitivity than wild-type obese mice despite no differences in body weight, fat mass, or adipose tissue inflammation.[50] In humans, insulin-stimulated glucose disposal is strongly correlated with insulin-suppressed FFA concentrations/flux,[51,52] and nadir FFA concentrations in response to intravenous glucose and meals are independent predictors of insulin sensitivity.[53] These data support the concept that dysregulation of adipose tissue lipolysis, including reduced ability of insulin to suppress FFA, may precede and cause muscle and liver insulin resistance. Furthermore, upper-body subcutaneous adipose tissue is the major source of these FFA.[33,43] What is the reason for dysregulation of subcutaneous adipose tissue in humans predisposed to visceral obesity?

ASSOCIATION BETWEEN VISCERAL FAT AND DYSREGULATION OF SUBCUTANEOUS ADIPOSE DYSFUNCTION

Dr Danforth most clearly stated the hypothesis that abnormalities of subcutaneous fat were at the heart of the visceral obesity/insulin resistance/type 2 diabetes phenomenon in 2000.[54] He posited that the hypertrophic nature of abdominal subcutaneous adipocytes in those predisposed to type 2 diabetes could be explained by a failure of preadipocytes to differentiate in response to the need for additional body fat expansion. Hypertrophic adipocytes have excess rates of lipolysis and are insulin resistant. **Fig. 1** depicts the relative extremes of potential fat gain, ranging from a fat storage solely into hypertrophic subcutaneous adipocytes (lower left) with substantial gain of visceral fat to excess fat storage solely from hyperplasia, with maintenance of normal subcutaneous fat cell size and function (lower right) and little gain of visceral fat.

Since Dr Danforth's original commentary, there has been remarkable progress in understanding the factors that drive adipogenesis.[55] An excellent review of the nature

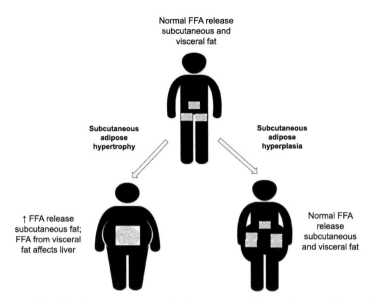

Fig. 1. Gain of body fat by storing excess fat in new, normal size adipocytes (hyperplasia) is associated with maintenance of normal regulation of FFA release from adipose tissue lipolysis. People who gain fat via this process tend to have a predominantly lower-body fat distribution. Gain of body fat by storing excess fat in ever larger adipocytes (hypertrophy) is associated with excess FFA release and storage of fat in visceral fat and ectopic depots. Hypertrophic obesity often presents as preferential upper-body fat gain. In this type of obesity, the liver is adversely affected by excess FFA from both subcutaneous and visceral fat, whereas all other tissues are exposed to FFA coming predominantly from dysregulated subcutaneous adipose tissue. Visceral fat gain appears to be the result of dysfunctional subcutaneous adipose tissue, not the cause of dysfunctional subcutaneous adipose tissue.

of hypertrophic obesity and the cellular/molecular mechanisms that are behind this phenotype has recently been published.[56] The main points of these investigators are that those for whom subcutaneous adipose tissue has a limited ability to expand owing to defects in recruiting precursor cells to proliferate and/or differentiate (leading to enlarged size of existing adipocytes), and it is likely that epigenetic and genetic factors regulate adipogenesis. They suggest that bone morphogenetic protein-4 and its endogenous antagonist gremlin-1 are key factors that might link together the complex phenomena of adipose tissue proliferation and differentiation. Defects in these processes, whether inherited or acquired, may explain the tendency of some humans to gain body fat predominantly by adipocyte hypertrophy, with its attendant problems, as opposed to hyperplasia.

A reasonable interpretation of this information is that those humans with defects in the ability of adipocyte precursors to proliferate and differentiate in response to the need for more fat storage develop dysfunctional subcutaneous adipocytes, which expose peripheral tissues to excess FFA. In addition, these excess FFA drive the storage of fat in ectopic depots, including visceral fat, liver, intramyocellular triglycerides, pericardial fat, and the adipose tissue seen as marbling in muscle. Evidence for this theory comes from an overfeeding study that reported adults who gain more fat via creation of new leg adipocytes are protected from visceral fat gain compared with those who gain fat more so by increasing adipocyte size in abdominal subcutaneous fat.[57]

SUMMARY

Although there is no question that excess amounts of visceral fat are strongly associated with several metabolic abnormalities, only a subset of these are likely to be a direct result of dysfunction of visceral fat. These abnormalities include hypertriglyceridemia, increases in CRP, and possibly hepatic insulin resistance with regards to suppression of glucose production. The most likely cause of excess visceral fat gain seems to be the forced storage of fatty acids, possibly from excess fasting and postprandial FFA release, as a result of insulin resistant subcutaneous fat. Insulin resistance in subcutaneous fat in turn can be attributed to expansion of upper-body subcutaneous adipose tissue by adipocyte hypertrophy rather than hyperplasia. Excess systemic FFA from subcutaneous adipose tissue lipolysis directly impacts all peripheral tissues and even liver to a significant extent.[33] Thus, interpretation of the available literature suggests that expansion of visceral fat is in large part canary and only in small part culprit when it comes to metabolic illnesses.

DISCLOSURE

This work was supported by National Institutes of Health Grants DK45343 and DK40484. The content is solely the responsibility of the author and does not necessarily represent the official views of the National Institutes of Health.

REFERENCES

1. Kissebah AH, Alfarsi S, Adams PW, et al. Role of insulin resistance in adipose tissue and liver in the pathogenesis of endogenous hypertriglyceridaemia in man. Diabetologia 1976;12:563–71.
2. Cassano PA, Segel MR, Vokonas PS, et al. Body fat distribution, blood pressure, and hypertension. A prospective cohort study of men in the normative aging study. Ann Epidemiol 1990;1(1):33–48.
3. Seidell JC, Cigolini M, Deslypere J, et al. Body fat distribution in relation to serum lipids and blood pressure in 38-year-old European men: the European fat distribution study. Atherosclerosis 1991;86:251–60.
4. Carey VJ, Walters EE, Colditz GA, et al. Body fat distribution and risk of non-insulin dependent diabetes mellitus in women. Am J Epidemiol 1997;145:614–9.
5. Chan JM, Rimm EB, Colditz GA, et al. Obesity, fat distribution, and weight gain as risk factors for clinical diabetes in men. Diabetes Care 1994;17(9):961–9.
6. Snijder MB, Dekker JM, Visser M, et al. Trunk fat and leg fat have independent and opposite associations with fasting and postload glucose levels: the Hoorn study. Diabetes Care 2004;27(2):372–7.
7. Cefalu WT, Wang ZQ, Webel S, et al. Contribution of visceral fat mass to the insulin resistance of aging. Metabolism 1995;44:954–9.
8. Seidell JC, Bjorntorp P, Sjostrom L, et al. Visceral fat accumulation in men is positively associated with insulin, glucose, and C-peptide levels, but negatively with testosterone levels. Metabolism 1990;39(9):897–901.
9. Kuk JL, Katzmarzyk PT, Nichaman MZ, et al. Visceral fat is an independent predictor of all-cause mortality in men. Obesity (Silver Spring) 2006;14(2):336–42.
10. Abate N, Garg A, Peshock RM, et al. Relationships of generalized and regional adiposity to insulin sensitivity in men. J Clin Invest 1995;96:88–98.
11. Kelley DE, Thaete FL, Troost F, et al. Subdivisions of subcutaneous abdominal adipose tissue and insulin resistance. Am J Physiol 2000;278:E941–8.

12. Smith SR, Lovejoy JC, Greenway F, et al. Contributions of total body fat, abdominal subcutaneous adipose tissue compartments, and visceral adipose tissue to the metabolic complications of obesity. Metabolism 2001;50(4):425–35.

13. Tchoukalova YD, Koutsari C, Karpyak MV, et al. Subcutaneous adipocyte size and body fat distribution. Am J Clin Nutr 2008;87:56–63.

14. Goodpaster BH, Thaete FL, Kelley DE. Thigh adipose tissue distribution is associated with insulin resistance in obesity and in type 2 diabetes mellitus. Am J Clin Nutr 2000;71(4):885–92.

15. Richelsen B, Pedersen SB, Moller-Pedersen T, et al. Regional differences in triglyceride breakdown in human adipose tissue: effects of catecholamines, insulin, and prostaglandin E2. Metabolism 1991;40:990–6.

16. Arner P, Hellstrom L, Wahrenberg H, et al. Beta-adrenoceptor expression in human fat cells from different regions. J Clin Invest 1990;86:1595–600.

17. Arner P, Kriegholm E, Engfeldt P. In situ studies of catecholamine-induced lipolysis in human adipose tissue using microdialysis. J Pharmacol Exp Ther 1990; 254:284–8.

18. Marin P, Andersson B, Ottosson M, et al. The morphology and metabolism of intraabdominal adipose tissue in men. Metabolism 1992;41:1242–8.

19. Votruba SB, Jensen MD. Sex-specific differences in leg fat uptake are revealed with a high-fat meal. Am J Physiol 2006;291:E1115–23.

20. Votruba SB, Mattison RS, Dumesic DA, et al. Meal fatty acid uptake in visceral fat in women. Diabetes 2007;56:2589–97.

21. Ibrahim MM. Subcutaneous and visceral adipose tissue: structural and functional differences. Obes Rev 2010;11(1):11–8.

22. Jensen MD, Kanaley JA, Reed JE, et al. Measurement of abdominal and visceral fat with computed tomography and dual-energy x-ray absorptiometry. Am J Clin Nutr 1995;61:274–8.

23. Shadid S, Jensen MD. Effects of pioglitazone vs diet and exercise on metabolic health and fat distribution in upper body obesity. Diabetes Care 2003;26: 3148–52.

24. Harman-Boehm I, Bluher M, Redel H, et al. Macrophage infiltration into omental versus subcutaneous fat across different populations: effect of regional adiposity and the comorbidities of obesity. J Clin Endocrinol Metab 2007;92(6):2240–7.

25. Tchkonia T, Zhu Y, van Deursen J, et al. Cellular senescence and the senescent secretory phenotype: therapeutic opportunities. J Clin Invest 2012;123(3): 966–72.

26. Despres JP. Abdominal obesity as important component of insulin-resistance syndrome. Nutrition 1993;9(5):452–9.

27. Goodpaster BH, Thaete FL, Simoneau JA, et al. Subcutaneous abdominal fat and thigh muscle composition predict insulin sensitivity independently of visceral fat. Diabetes 1997;46(10):1579–85.

28. Banerji M, Faridi N, Atluri R, et al. Body composition, visceral fat, leptin, and insulin resistance in Asian Indian men. J Clin Endocrinol Metab 1999;84:137–44.

29. Banerji MA, Lebowitz J, Chaiken RL, et al. Relationship of visceral adipose tissue and glucose disposal is independent of sex in black NIDDM subjects. Am J Physiol 1997;273(2 Pt 1):E425–32.

30. Miyazaki Y, Glass L, Triplitt C, et al. Abdominal fat distribution and peripheral and hepatic insulin resistance in type 2 diabetes mellitus. Am J Physiol 2002;283: E1135–43.

31. Lewis GF, Uffelman KD, Szeto LW, et al. Interaction between free fatty acids and insulin in the acute control of very low density lipoprotein production in humans. J Clin Invest 1995;95:158–66.
32. Ostman J, Arner P, Engfeldt P, et al. Regional differences in the control of lipolysis in human adipose tissue. Metabolism 1979;28(12):1198–205.
33. Nielsen S, Guo ZK, Johnson CM, et al. Splanchnic lipolysis in human obesity. J Clin Invest 2004;113(11):1582–8.
34. Basu A, Basu R, Shah P, et al. Systemic and regional free fatty acid metabolism in type 2 diabetes. Am J Physiol 2001;280:E1000–6.
35. Vogelberg KH, Gries FA, Moschinski D. Hepatic production of VLDL-triglycerides. Dependence of portal substrate and insulin concentration. Horm Metab Res 1980;12:688–94.
36. Fontana L, Eagon JC, Trujillo ME, et al. Visceral fat adipokine secretion is associated with systemic inflammation in obese humans. Diabetes 2007;56(4):1010–3.
37. Mohamed-Ali V, Goodrick S, Rawesh A, et al. Subcutaneous adipose tissue releases interleukin-6, but not tumor necrosis factor-alpha, in vivo. J Clin Endocrinol Metab 1997;82(12):4196–200.
38. Marin P, Oden B, Olbe L, et al. Assimilation of triglycerides in subcutaneous and intraabdominal adipose tissues in vivo in men: effects of testosterone. J Clin Endocrinol Metab 1996;81:1018–22.
39. Sondergaard E, Nellemann B, Sorensen LP, et al. Similar VLDL-TG storage in visceral and subcutaneous fat in obese and lean women. Diabetes 2011;60:2787–91.
40. Ali AH, Koutsari C, Mundi M, et al. Free fatty acid storage in human visceral and subcutaneous adipose tissue: role of adipocyte proteins. Diabetes 2011;60:2300–7.
41. Bucci M, Karmi AC, Iozzo P, et al. Enhanced fatty acid uptake in visceral adipose tissue is not reversed by weight loss in obese individuals with the metabolic syndrome. Diabetologia 2015;58(1):158–64.
42. Roust LR, Jensen MD. Postprandial free fatty acid kinetics are abnormal in upper body obesity. Diabetes 1993;42:1567–73.
43. Guo ZK, Hensrud DD, Johnson CM, et al. Regional postprandial fatty acid metabolism in different obesity phenotypes. Diabetes 1999;48:1586–92.
44. Boden G, Chen X, Ruiz J, et al. Mechanisms of fatty acid-induced inhibition of glucose uptake. J Clin Invest 1994;93:2438–46.
45. Boden G, Jadali F. Effects of lipid on basal carbohydrate metabolism in normal men. Diabetes 1991;40:686–92.
46. Boden G, Lebed B, Schatz M, et al. Effects of acute changes of plasma free fatty acids on intramyocellular fat content and insulin resistance in healthy subjects. Diabetes 2001;50:1612–7.
47. Roden M, Price TB, Perseghin G, et al. Mechanism of free fatty acid-induced insulin resistance in humans. J Clin Invest 1996;97(12):2859–65.
48. Saloranta C, Franssila-Kallunki A, Ekstrand A, et al. Modulation of hepatic glucose production by non-esterified fatty acids in type 2 (non-insulin-dependent) diabetes mellitus. Diabetologia 1991;34:409–15.
49. Bajaj M, Suraamornkul S, Kashyap S, et al. Sustained reduction in plasma free fatty acid concentration improves insulin action without altering plasma adipocytokine levels in subjects with strong family history of type 2 diabetes. J Clin Endocrinol Metab 2004;89(9):4649–55.

50. Girousse A, Tavernier G, Valle C, et al. Partial inhibition of adipose tissue lipolysis improves glucose metabolism and insulin sensitivity without alteration of fat mass. PLoS Biol 2013;11(2):e1001485.

51. Magkos F, Fabbrini E, Conte C, et al. Relationship between adipose tissue lipolytic activity and skeletal muscle insulin resistance in nondiabetic women. J Clin Endocrinol Metab 2012;97(7):E1219–23.

52. Shadid S, Kanaley JA, Sheehan MT, et al. Basal and insulin-regulated free fatty acid and glucose metabolism in humans. Am J Physiol 2007;292:E1770–4.

53. Bush NC, Basu R, Rizza RA, et al. Insulin-mediated FFA suppression is associated with triglyceridemia and insulin sensitivity independent of adiposity. J Clin Endocrinol Metab 2012;97(11):4130–8.

54. Danforth E Jr. Failure of adipocyte differentiation causes type II diabetes mellitus? Nat Genet 2000;26:13.

55. Hammarstedt A, Graham TE, Kahn BB. Adipose tissue dysregulation and reduced insulin sensitivity in non-obese individuals with enlarged abdominal adipose cells. Diabetol Metab Syndr 2012;4(1):42.

56. Hammarstedt A, Gogg S, Hedjazifar S, et al. Impaired adipogenesis and dysfunctional adipose tissue in human hypertrophic obesity. Physiol Rev 2018; 98(4):1911–41.

57. Tchoukalova Y, Votruba SB, Tchkonia T, et al. Regional differences in cellular mechanisms of adipose tissue gain with overfeeding. Proc Natl Acad Sci U S A 2010;107:18226–31.

Growth Hormone and Obesity

Astrid Hjelholt, MD, PhD[a,b], Morten Høgild, MD[a,b], Ann Mosegaard Bak, MD[a,b], Mai Christiansen Arlien-Søborg, MD[a,b], Amanda Bæk, MD[a,b], Niels Jessen, MD[c,d,e], Bjørn Richelsen, MD[a,b,c], Steen Bønløkke Pedersen, MD[a,b], Niels Møller, MD[a,b], Jens Otto Lunde Jørgensen, MD[a,b],*

KEYWORDS

- Growth hormone • Insulin-like growth factor I • Obesity

KEY POINTS

- Growth hormone induces protein anabolism via stimulation of insulin-like growth factor-I production and fat catabolism via direct lipolytic effects in adipose tissue.
- The anabolic effect depends on a positive energy balance and portal insulin levels, whereas the lipolytic effect prevails in the postabsorptive and fasting states.
- Obesity is characterized by reversible suppression of growth hormone secretion driven by elevated free fatty acid levels and normal serum insulin-like growth factor-I levels.
- The physiologic response to fasting is less pronounced in obesity and may represent a compensatory mechanism to dampen fasting-induced insulin resistance and preserve lean body mass.
- Activation of the growth hormone axis as an adjunct treatment of obesity has so far proven of limited therapeutic use.

INTRODUCTION

Growth hormone (GH) is a peptide hormone secreted from the pituitary gland with pleiotropic metabolic effects.[1,2] It is essential for induction of postnatal longitudinal growth and this effect is predominantly mediated by the GH-induced production and anabolic action of insulin-like growth factor I (IGF-I).[3] However, it was recognized early that GH also regulates substrate metabolism and, in particular, potently

a Medical Research Laboratory, Department of Clinical Medicine, Aarhus University Hospital, Aarhus N 8200, Denmark; b Medical Research Laboratory, Department of Endocrinology and Internal Medicine, Aarhus University Hospital, Aarhus N 8200, Denmark; c Steno Diabetes Center Aarhus, Aarhus University Hospital, Palle Juul-Jensens Boulevard 99, Aarhus 8200, Denmark; d Department of Clinical Pharmacology, Aarhus University Hospital, Aarhus, Denmark; e Department of Biomedicine, Aarhus University, Aarhus, Denmark
* Corresponding author. Department of Endocrinology and Internal Medicine, Aarhus University Hospital, Palle Juul-Jensens Boulevard 99, Aarhus N 8200, Denmark.
E-mail address: joj@clin.au.dk

stimulates lipolysis.[4] This effect is independent of IGF-I and predominantly operates in the postabsorptive and fasting states.[5]

The anabolic and lipolytic effects of GH translate into changes in body composition as exemplified by the phenotype of active acromegaly, a condition caused by GH hypersecretion from a benign pituitary adenoma, which is characterized by reduced fat mass and increased lean body mass.[6] Moreover, adult patients with GH deficiency are moderately obese and this stTE reverses by GH replacement.[7] Last but not least, GH secretion is blunted in obese patients.[8]

Taken together, GH status is a potential determinant of obesity and hence the topic of this review, which focuses on studies in human subjects.

GROWTH HORMONE SECRETION IN OBESITY

The advent of reliable immunologic methods to measure circulating hormones was an important milestone that revealed a pulsatile GH pattern.[9] The regulation of GH secretion is complex and beyond the scope of this review,[10] but suffice it to say that obesity blunts the GH response to hypoglycemia as well as to arginine stimulation.[8,11] We later documented that intra-abdominal fat even in clinically nonobese healthy persons is a very strong negative determinant of GH secretion.[12] These associations have led to the speculation that impaired GH secretion could be a primary or even causal attribute of obesity, but intended massive weight loss normalizes GH secretion in obesity,[13] which suggests that blunted GH secretion is an effect rather than a cause of obesity. Of note, total serum IGF-I levels are not decrease in obesity; in fact, bioactive IGF-I levels are even slightly elevated as compared with normal weight subjects.[14] This paradox may be explained by the elevated insulin levels in obesity, because portal insulin per se promotes hepatic IGF-I production and at the same time suppresses the formation of IGF-binding protein 1.[15] Thus, an increase in free and bioactive IGF-I sustained by insulin could explain the suppressed GH secretion via negative feedback mechanisms.

It is also plausible that the elevation in free fatty acids (FFA) that accompanies obesity contributes to GH suppression, because circulating FFAs inhibit GH secretion, whereas experimental lowering of FFA levels reverses obesity-associated impairment of GH secretion.[16] Taken together, it can be hypothesized that (1) obesity induces feedback inhibition of pituitary GH secretion predominantly via increased nonfasting serum FFA levels, (2) the associated insulin resistance causes a compensatory increase in portal insulin levels that stimulates IGF-I production and suppresses IGF-binding protein 1 production, and (3) the net result is blunted GH levels but normal IGF-I levels (**Fig. 1**). Irrespective of the underlying mechanisms, low GH levels may contribute to maintenance of the obese state and GH administration or activation of endogenous GH secretion as a treatment for obesity has been tested, as discussed elsewhere in this article.

GROWTH HORMONE SIGNALING AND ACTION IN HUMAN ADIPOSE TISSUE
Early Metabolic Studies

Maurice Raben stated 60 years ago that the increase in FFA was "perhaps the most sensitive response to GH of any yet described."[17] Consistent with the lipolytic action, serum GH levels were later shown to be suppressed after meals and elevated during fasting.[18] Rabinowitz and Zierler[19] used these observations and performed experimental studies on the metabolic in vivo effects of GH and insulin in human subjects. They demonstrated that GH stimulates lipolysis in adipose tissue, leading to the uptake and oxidation of FFA in skeletal muscle. They also showed that GH acutely

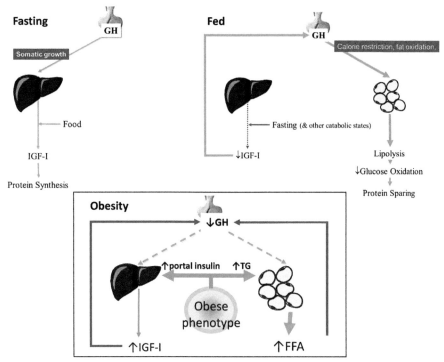

Fig. 1. Regulation and action of GH as a function of substrate background. In the presence of a positive energy balance (fed), GH induces protein anabolism mainly mediated by IGF-I. During fasting, IGF-I production is suppressed, which contributes to the feedback stimulation of GH secretion and GH-induced stimulation of lipolysis. In manifest obesity, sustained FFA levels feedback inhibits pituitary GH secretion, but IGF-I levels are normal or even slightly elevated owing to a stimulatory effect of portal insulin on hepatic IGF-I production.

and directly induces resistance to insulin-stimulated glucose uptake in skeletal muscle.[19] Because the circulating pattern of insulin are reciprocal to that of GH, they hypothesized the following: (1) immediately after a meal, insulin acts alone to promote the storage of glucose and other nutrients, (2) in the fasting state, GH acts alone to promote mobilization and oxidation of endogenous lipid stores, and (3) between these 2 phases, GH and insulin act in synergy to promote protein anabolism.[5] This hypothesis has stood the test of time; indeed, the subsequent discovery of IGF-I as a GH-dependent protein anabolic peptide fits well in, because portal insulin levels stimulate hepatic IGF-I formation and elevate free IGF-I levels via suppression of IGF-binding protein 1 formation (**Fig. 2**).

Growth Hormone Signaling

GH binds to a preformed receptor (GH receptor [GHR]) dimer, leading to a conformational GHR change that initiates JAK2-STAT5 phosphorylation. Phosphorylated and dimerized STAT proteins translocate to the nucleus, where they bind to gamma-activated site motifs to regulate GH target genes.[20] Independent of JAK2, GH binding to the GHR also leads to autophosphorylation of Src kinase that phosphorylates protein kinase C and activates the extracellular signal regulated kinases (ERK1/2) and MAPK signaling pathways.[20] We have consistently demonstrated that systemic GH acutely

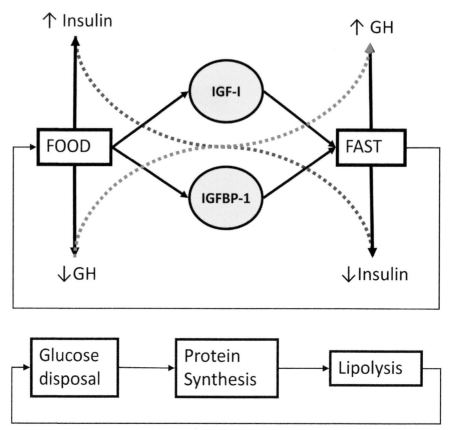

Fig. 2. Schematic illustration of the feast–famine (food–fast) cycle hypothesis. In the post-prandial period (FOOD), insulin levels are high and GH levels low, favoring insulin-induced disposal of nutrients. In the postabsorptive or fasting state (FAST), GH is elevated and insulin low, favoring GH-induced lipolysis. In the intermediate period, insulin and IGF-I act in synergy to promote protein anabolism.

activates the JAK-STAT5 signaling pathway in human adipose tissue in vivo, whereas we have been unable to record consistent activation of the MAPK pathway.[21–25]

Because obese individuals exhibit normal (or even slightly elevated) serum IGF-I levels in the presence of blunted GH secretion, it could be hypothesized that GH sensitivity or responsiveness is increased at the level of GH signaling. This finding is, however, not supported by the observation of decreased GHR messenger RNA (mRNA) expression in subcutaneous and omental fat from obese subjects.[26] Likewise, we have shown that GH signaling and action do not differ between obese and lean subjects in a study assessing STAT5 phosphorylation and mRNA expression of canonical target genes (*igf1* and *SOCS/CISH*) in adipose tissue in vivo after acute GH exposure.[27]

Regulation of Lipolysis

Lipolysis is the metabolic pathway through which triglyceride (TG) is hydrolyzed into 1 glycerol and 3 fatty acids coordinated by a number of proteins including enzymes and lipid droplet-associated proteins[28] **(Fig. 3)**.

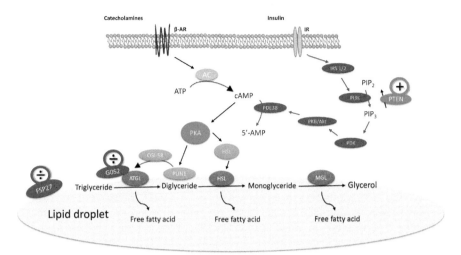

Fig. 3. Simplified illustration of the regulation of lipolysis in adipose tissue. GH has been shown to downregulate the expression of G0S2 and FSP27 both of which act as suppressors of lipolysis, and to upregulate phosphatase and tensin homolog (PTEN), which suppresses insulin-induced antilipolysis. Thus, GH mainly promotes lipolysis via suppression of antilipolytic signals.

It involves the sequential action of 3 lipases: adipose TG lipase (ATGL), hormone-sensitive lipase, and monoacylglycerol lipase, of which ATGL is the rate-limiting enzyme that catalyzes hydrolysis of TG to diacylglycerol.[29] Perilipin A is a lipid droplet protein that inhibits ATGL activity by preventing its interaction with comparative gene identification-58. Protein kinase A activation phosphorylates perilipin A, which releases comparative gene identification-5, which then binds to and stimulates ATGL. Translocation of ATGL to lipid droplets, along with phosphorylated hormone-sensitive lipase, leads to acute activation of TG hydrolysis.[29]

ATGL activity is negatively regulated by G0S2 G0/G1 Switch 2 (G0S2) and fat-specific protein 27. G0S2 binds directly to ATGL and attenuates ATGL-mediated lipolysis by inhibiting its enzymatic activity.[30] Fat-specific protein 27 is a lipid droplet protein that inhibits both the activity and expression of ATGL.[31,32]

The primary stimulator of lipolysis is β-adrenergic receptor-mediated cAMP formation that activates protein kinase A, whereas insulin is the major inhibitor of lipolysis via Akt-dependent suppression of cAMP and protein kinase A activity.

The molecular mechanisms whereby GH stimulates lipolysis in human subjects in vivo are not yet fully settled, but it is completely blocked by acipimox, a nicotinic acid derivative.[33–35] Acipimox binds to the hydroxyl-carboxylic acid receptor 2 (HCA$_2$, alias GPR109a and HM74a), which is coupled to G$_i$-type G proteins, on adipocytes, and suppresses cAMP formation.[36] The endogenous ligand of HCA$_2$ is the ketone body 3-hydroxy-butyrate.[36]

More recently, we have shown that GH-induced lipolysis in healthy human subjects includes suppression of fat-specific protein 27 expression,[37] as well as suppression of G0S2 mRNA expression.[38] In the latter study, we also recorded upregulation of phosphatase and tensin homolog mRNA expression, which acts to suppress insulin signaling.

These human in vivo effects of GH on lipolytic regulators were accompanied by STAT5 signaling, including upregulation of CISH and IGF-I mRNA, whereas no evidence of MAPK signaling has been recorded, but the latter could reflect the methodologic limitations inherent to human in vivo studies. A study showed that GH-induced lipolysis in adipose tissue is STAT5 mediated in mice,[39,40] but there are data from in vitro and mouse studies to suggest a dependence on Src kinase-MAPK signaling.[37,41,42]

Regardless of the GH signaling mechanism, the human data collected so far indicate that the lipolytic effects of GH in human adipose tissue in vivo mainly comprise suppression of antilipolysis, that is, a release of the brakes, rather than activation of the accelerator (see **Fig. 3**).

Regulation of Lipoprotein Lipase Activity in Adipose Tissue

Circulating TG bound to lipoproteins are taken up in peripheral tissues as FFA catalyzed by the lipoprotein lipase (LPL), which is attached to the luminal side of the endothelium. In adipose tissue, FFAs are predominantly re-esterified into TG for storage,[43,44] whereas in skeletal muscle, LPL promotes FFA uptake as a fuel for oxidation.[45] LPL activity is negatively regulated by angiopoietin-like protein 4 (ANGPTL4),[46] which is upregulated by fasting and suppressed by food intake and insulin.[47–49]

GH suppresses LPL activity in human adipose tissue in vivo[50–52] and also upregulates *ANGPTL4* mRNA expression in skeletal muscle in human subjects in vivo via an FFA-dependent mechanism,[53] which is in accordance with data showing that plasma ANGPTL4 levels are increased by FFA.[46,54] The impact of GH on LPL activity in skeletal muscle is less studied, but a suppressive effect of exogenous GH as compared with placebo was reported after 5 weeks of weight loss induced by a hypocaloric diet in obese women.[51]

GROWTH HORMONE IN RESPONSE TO FASTING IN OBESE SUBJECTS

Fasting triggers a hormonally driven metabolic adaptation aimed at ensuring energy use from lipid stores and thereby limiting the need for gluconeogenesis from protein breakdown.[55] Most, but not all, tissues can use FFA via β-oxidation, whereas the brain initially relies on glucose derived from gluconeogenesis. More prolonged fasting stimulates ketogenesis, which is used in the brain.[55] Fasting also induces insulin resistance, which contributes to glucose sparing.[56] This finding is corroborated by suppressed insulin levels in concomitance with amplified secretion and action of counter-regulatory hormones. The counter-regulatory response includes stimulation of GH secretion,[57] triggered by a reduction in serum IGF-I levels.[58]

Because weight loss and hence a negative energy balance is the pivotal component of any obesity treatment, it is of obvious relevance to study the GH response to fasting in obese individuals. In this regard, experimental data in obese individuals yield conflicting results regarding GH and IGF-I levels in response to fasting.[59,60] In a recent study, we compared substrate metabolism and GH status in 9 obese and 9 normal weight individuals before and after a 72-hour fast.[27] As expected, GH levels in the obese group were blunted but increased in response to fasting to the same relative degree (percent increase from baseline) as compared with the normal weight group (approximately 5- to 6-fold increase in both groups.[27] Moreover, the response to a single exogenous GH bolus was comparable in terms of GH signaling in adipose tissue and induction of lipolysis and peripheral insulin resistance.[27] Of note, a GH-induced insulin-antagonistic effect on endogenous glucose production only occurred in the obese group. Moreover, a pronounced fasting-induced decrease in IGF-I levels occurred in the normal weight group, whereas a small increase was recorded in the obese group. Taken together, it was hypothesized that obesity confers increased sensitivity to the hepatic actions of GH (IGF-I production and suppression of endogenous glucose production). This notion is backed up by another recent study in obese individuals where GH blockade as compared with placebo decreased IGF-I levels as well as endogenous glucose production during a 36-hour fast.[61]

GROWTH HORMONE TREATMENT IN OBESITY

Considering the ability of GH to induce lipid catabolism and protein anabolism, it is perhaps not surprising that GH has been tested as a treatment of obesity.[62] In a meta-analysis including placebo-controlled trials, 24 studies were identified including almost 500 obese individuals being treated for on average about 12 weeks (range, 3–72 weeks).[62] Fat mass decreased by approximately 1 kg and lean body mass increased by approximately 2 kg associated with side effects in terms of transient elevations in plasma glucose and insulin and more sustained complaints of arthralgia and fluid retention.[62]

DISCUSSION

GH secretion is reversibly suppressed in obesity in the presence of normal IGF-I levels. This state is sustained by elevated FFA levels that inhibit pituitary GH secretion, and by elevated portal insulin levels that enhance hepatic IGF-I production and hence serum IGF-I levels. To which degree this unique pattern worsens the obese state or constitutes a favorable adaptation remains an open question. It is easy to argue that low GH levels blunts the lipolytic response to fasting and exercise and thereby impedes fat loss via these strategies. In contrast, low GH levels seem to dampen obesity-associated (FFA-driven) insulin resistance, whereas elevated GH levels would do the opposite and thereby compromise insulin-mediated substrate switching (metabolic inflexibility).

The lipolytic effects of GH are expressed in the postabsorptive and fasting state where endogenous GH levels in normal weight individuals are stimulated, which is triggered by decreased hepatic IGF-I production. From a teleologic point of view, this state constitutes a favorable adaptation (metabolic flexibility) that ensures oxidation of fatty acids and ketone bodies at the expense of glucose oxidation, which provides energy to the brain and protects the organism from excessive protein catabolism. This adaptive GH response to fasting is decreased in obese individuals, but the pathophysiologic implications are less clear. In a recent study where we compared the response to 72-hour fasting in obese (body mass index of approximately 36 kg/m^2) versus lean (body mass index of approximately 21 kg/m^2) individuals, a comparable absolute weight loss of approximately 4 kg was obtained.[63] Whole body lipolysis expressed as palmitate flux was higher after fasting in obese subjects, whereas palmitate flux per unit fat mass was reduced in obesity in response to fasting.[27] In addition, muscle protein breakdown across the forearm as well as urea flux and urinary nitrogen excretion were decreased during fasting as compared with the normal weight individuals.[27] As a part of the same study, we recorded blunted basal GH levels in the obese individuals, whereas fasting induced the same relative increase in serum GH levels in the obese subejcts.[27] Serum IGF-I levels declined significantly during fasting in the lean individuals but remained stable in the obese; interestingly, the IGF-I area under the curve during fasting correlated negatively with phenylalanine flux (a measure of protein loss) and positively with phenylalanine balance during fasting (**Fig. 4**). These associations strongly suggest a protective effect of IGF-I against protein loss during

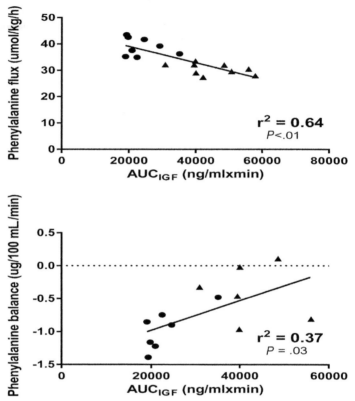

Fig. 4. Correlations between serum IGF-I levels and whole body phenylalanine flux AUC$_{IGF-I}$ and phenylalanine forearm balance per 100 mL tissue, respectively after 72 hours of fasting in obese (▲) and lean (●) subjects. The data are based on data from a previously published study AUC, area under the curve. (*Data from* Hogild ML, Bak AM, Pedersen SB, et al. Growth hormone signaling and action in obese versus lean human subjects. Am J Physiol Endocrinol Metab. 2019;316(2):E333-E344; and Pedersen MH, Svart MV, Lebeck J, et al. Substrate metabolism and insulin sensitivity during fasting in obese human subjects: Impact of GH Blockade. J Clin Endocrinol Metab. 2017;102(4):1340-1349.)

fasting and likely contributes to the observed relative preservation of lean body mass during fasting in the obese individuals.[63]

GH treatment of obese individuals has been tested in placebo-controlled trials, but has proven disappointing from a therapeutic point of view.[62]

Taken together, the physiologic and pathophysiologic implications of the altered GH–IGF-I axis in obesity remain uncertain, but GH is neither the cause nor the cure of obesity. Still, numerous original observations have been made that contributes to our understanding of the endocrine regulation of substrate metabolism and insulin sensitivity. A negative energy balance obtained by dietary measures in combination with increased physical activity remains the cornerstone of obesity treatment. Whether or not activation of the GH–IGF-I axis as adjunct therapy is useful remains uncertain.

DISCLOSURE

The authors have nothing to disclose in relation to this work.

REFERENCES

1. Jorgensen JO. Human growth hormone replacement therapy: pharmacological and clinical aspects. Endocr Rev 1991;12(3):189–207.
2. Moller N, Jorgensen JO. Effects of growth hormone on glucose, lipid, and protein metabolism in human subjects. Endocr Rev 2009;30(2):152–77.
3. Le Roith D, Bondy C, Yakar S, et al. The somatomedin hypothesis: 2001. Endocr Rev 2001;22(1):53–74.
4. Raben MS, Hollenberg CH. Effect of growth hormone on plasma fatty acids. J Clin Invest 1959;38(3):484–8.
5. Rabinowitz D, Zierler KL. A metabolic regulating device based on the actions of human growth hormone and of insulin, singly and together, on the human forearm. Nature 1963;199:913–5.
6. Freda PU, Shen W, Heymsfield SB, et al. Lower visceral and subcutaneous but higher intermuscular adipose tissue depots in patients with growth hormone and insulin-like growth factor I excess due to acromegaly. J Clin Endocrinol Metab 2008;93(6):2334–43.
7. Jorgensen JO, Vahl N, Hansen TB, et al. Growth hormone versus placebo treatment for one year in growth hormone deficient adults: increase in exercise capacity and normalization of body composition. Clin Endocrinol (Oxf) 1996;45(6): 681–8.
8. Copinschi G, Wegienka LC, Hane S, et al. Effect of arginine on serum levels of insulin and growth hormone in obese subjects. Metab Clin Exp 1967;16(6): 485–91.
9. Glick SM, Roth J, Yalow RS, et al. Immunoassay of human growth hormone in plasma. Nature 1963;199:784–7.
10. Giustina A, Veldhuis JD. Pathophysiology of the neuroregulation of growth hormone secretion in experimental animals and the human*. Endocr Rev 1998; 19(6):717–97.
11. Beck P, Koumans JH, Winterling CA, et al. Studies of insulin and growth hormone secretion in human obesity. J Lab Clin Med 1964;64:654–67.
12. Vahl N, Jorgensen JO, Skjaerbaek C, et al. Abdominal adiposity rather than age and sex predicts mass and regularity of GH secretion in healthy adults. Am J Physiol 1997;272(6 Pt 1):E1108–16.
13. Rasmussen MH, Hvidberg A, Juul A, et al. Massive weight loss restores 24-hour growth hormone release profiles and serum insulin-like growth factor-I levels in obese subjects. J Clin Endocrinol Metab 1995;80(4):1407–15.
14. Frystyk J, Brick DJ, Gerweck AV, et al. Bioactive insulin-like growth factor-I in obesity. J Clin Endocrinol Metab 2009;94(8):3093–7.
15. Brismar K, Fernqvist-Forbes E, Wahren J, et al. Effect of insulin on the hepatic production of insulin-like growth factor-binding protein-1 (IGFBP-1), IGFBP-3, and IGF-I in insulin-dependent diabetes. J Clin Endocrinol Metab 1994;79(3): 872–8.
16. Cordido F, Peino R, Penalva A, et al. Impaired growth hormone secretion in obese subjects is partially reversed by acipimox-mediated plasma free fatty acid depression. J Clin Endocrinol Metab 1996;81(3):914–8.
17. Raben MS. Growth hormone. N Engl J Med 1962;266(1):31–5.
18. Roth J, Glick SM, Yalow RS, et al. Hypoglycemia: a potent stimulus to secretion of growth hormone. Science 1963;140(3570):987–8.
19. Zierler KL, Rabinowitz D. Roles of insulin and growth hormone, based on studies of forearm metabolism in man. Medicine 1963;42:385–402.

20. Lanning NJ, Carter-Su C. Recent advances in growth hormone signaling. Rev Endocr Metab Disord 2006;7(4):225–35.

21. Nielsen C, Gormsen LC, Jessen N, et al. Growth hormone signaling in vivo in human muscle and adipose tissue: impact of insulin, substrate background, and growth hormone receptor blockade. J Clin Endocrinol Metab 2008;93(7): 2842–50.

22. Clasen BF, Poulsen MM, Escande C, et al. Growth hormone signaling in muscle and adipose tissue of obese human subjects: associations with measures of body composition and interaction with resveratrol treatment. J Clin Endocrinol Metab 2014;99(12):E2565–73.

23. Jorgensen JO, Jessen N, Pedersen SB, et al. GH receptor signaling in skeletal muscle and adipose tissue in human subjects following exposure to an intravenous GH bolus. Am J Physiol Endocrinol Metab 2006;291(5):E899–905.

24. Moller L, Dalman L, Norrelund H, et al. Impact of fasting on growth hormone signaling and action in muscle and fat. J Clin Endocrinol Metab 2009;94(3): 965–72.

25. Vestergaard PF, Vendelbo MH, Pedersen SB, et al. GH signaling in skeletal muscle and adipose tissue in healthy human subjects: impact of gender and age. Eur J Endocrinol 2014;171(5):623–31.

26. Erman A, Veilleux A, Tchernof A, et al. Human growth hormone receptor (GHR) expression in obesity: I. GHR mRNA expression in omental and subcutaneous adipose tissues of obese women. Int J Obes (Lond) 2011;35(12):1511–9.

27. Hogild ML, Bak AM, Pedersen SB, et al. Growth hormone signaling and action in obese versus lean human subjects. Am J Physiol Endocrinol Metab 2019;316(2): E333–44.

28. Nielsen TS, Jessen N, Jorgensen JO, et al. Dissecting adipose tissue lipolysis: molecular regulation and implications for metabolic disease. J Mol Endocrinol 2014;52(3):R199–222.

29. Zechner R, Zimmermann R, Eichmann TO, et al. FAT SIGNALS–lipases and lipolysis in lipid metabolism and signaling. Cell Metab 2012;15(3):279–91.

30. Yang X, Lu X, Lombes M, et al. The G(0)/G(1) switch gene 2 regulates adipose lipolysis through association with adipose triglyceride lipase. Cell Metab 2010; 11(3):194–205.

31. Grahn TH, Kaur R, Yin J, et al. Fat-specific protein 27 (FSP27) interacts with adipose triglyceride lipase (ATGL) to regulate lipolysis and insulin sensitivity in human adipocytes. J Biol Chem 2014;289(17):12029–39.

32. Singh M, Kaur R, Lee MJ, et al. Fat-specific protein 27 inhibits lipolysis by facilitating the inhibitory effect of transcription factor Egr1 on transcription of adipose triglyceride lipase. J Biol Chem 2014;289(21):14481–7.

33. Nielsen S, Moller N, Christiansen JS, et al. Pharmacological antilipolysis restores insulin sensitivity during growth hormone exposure. Diabetes 2001;50(10): 2301–8.

34. Segerlantz M, Bramnert M, Manhem P, et al. Inhibition of the rise in FFA by Acipimox partially prevents GH-induced insulin resistance in GH-deficient adults. J Clin Endocrinol Metab 2001;86(12):5813–8.

35. Segerlantz M, Bramnert M, Manhem P, et al. Inhibition of lipolysis during acute GH exposure increases insulin sensitivity in previously untreated GH-deficient adults. Eur J Endocrinol 2003;149(6):511–9.

36. Offermanns S. Hydroxy-carboxylic acid receptor actions in metabolism. Trends Endocrinol Metab 2017;28(3):227–36.

37. Sharma VM, Vestergaard ET, Jessen N, et al. Growth hormone acts along the PPARgamma-FSP27 axis to stimulate lipolysis in human adipocytes. Am J Physiol Endocrinol Metab 2019;316(1):E34–42.
38. Hjelholt AJ, Lee KY, Arlien-Søborg MC, et al. Temporal patterns of lipolytic regulators in adipose tissue after acute growth hormone exposure in human subjects: a randomized controlled crossover trial. Mol Metab 2019;29:65–75.
39. Kaltenecker D, Mueller KM, Benedikt P, et al. Adipocyte STAT5 deficiency promotes adiposity and impairs lipid mobilisation in mice. Diabetologia 2017; 60(2):296–305.
40. Fain JN, Ihle JH, Bahouth SW. Stimulation of lipolysis but not of leptin release by growth hormone is abolished in adipose tissue from Stat5a and b knockout mice. Biochem Biophys Res Commun 1999;263(1):201–5.
41. Bergan HE, Kittilson JD, Sheridan MA. PKC and ERK mediate GH-stimulated lipolysis. J Mol Endocrinol 2013;51(2):213–24.
42. Sharma R, Luong Q, Sharma VM, et al. Growth hormone controls lipolysis by regulation of FSP27 expression. J Endocrinol 2018;239(3):289–301.
43. Santamarinafojo S, Brewer HB. Lipoprotein-lipase - structure, function and mechanism of action. Int J Clin Lab Res 1994;24(3):143–7.
44. Gutgsell AR, Ghodge SV, Bowers AA, et al. Mapping the sites of the lipoprotein lipase (LPL)-angiopoietin-like protein 4 (ANGPTL4) interaction provides mechanistic insight into LPL inhibition. J Biol Chem 2019;294(8):2678–89.
45. Kersten S. Physiological regulation of lipoprotein lipase. Biochim Biophys Acta 2014;1841(7):919–33.
46. Kersten S, Lichtenstein L, Steenbergen E, et al. Caloric restriction and exercise increase plasma ANGPTL4 levels in humans via elevated free fatty acids. Arterioscler Thromb Vasc Biol 2009;29(6):969–74.
47. Dijk W, Schutte S, Aarts EO, et al. Regulation of angiopoietin-like 4 and lipoprotein lipase in human adipose tissue. J Clin Lipidol 2018;12(3):773–83.
48. Dijk W, Kersten S. Regulation of lipoprotein lipase by Angptl4. Trends Endocrinol Metab 2014;25(3):146–55.
49. Cinkajzlova A, Mraz M, Lacinova Z, et al. Angiopoietin-like protein 3 and 4 in obesity, type 2 diabetes mellitus, and malnutrition: the effect of weight reduction and realimentation. Nutr Diabetes 2018;8(1):21.
50. Richelsen B, Pedersen SB, Borglum JD, et al. Growth hormone treatment of obese women for 5 wk: effect on body composition and adipose tissue LPL activity. Am J Physiol 1994;266(2 Pt 1):E211–6.
51. Richelsen B, Pedersen SB, Kristensen K, et al. Regulation of lipoprotein lipase and hormone-sensitive lipase activity and gene expression in adipose and muscle tissue by growth hormone treatment during weight loss in obese patients. Metab Clin Exp 2000;49(7):906–11.
52. Ottosson M, Vikman-Adolfsson K, Enerback S, et al. Growth hormone inhibits lipoprotein lipase activity in human adipose tissue. J Clin Endocrinol Metab 1995;80(3):936–41.
53. Clasen BF, Krusenstjerna-Hafstrom T, Vendelbo MH, et al. Gene expression in skeletal muscle after an acute intravenous GH bolus in human subjects: identification of a mechanism regulating ANGPTL4. J Lipid Res 2013;54(7):1988–97.
54. Brands M, Sauerwein HP, Ackermans MT, et al. Omega-3 long-chain fatty acids strongly induce angiopoietin-like 4 in humans. J Lipid Res 2013;54(3):615–21.
55. Cahill GF Jr. Fuel metabolism in starvation. Annu Rev Nutr 2006;26:1–22.
56. Vendelbo MH, Clasen BF, Treebak JT, et al. Insulin resistance after a 72-h fast is associated with impaired AS160 phosphorylation and accumulation of lipid and

glycogen in human skeletal muscle. Am J Physiol Endocrinol Metab 2012;302(2): E190–200.

57. Ho KY, Veldhuis JD, Johnson ML, et al. Fasting enhances growth hormone secretion and amplifies the complex rhythms of growth hormone secretion in man. J Clin Invest 1988;81(4):968–75.

58. Clemmons DR, Klibanski A, Underwood LE, et al. Reduction of plasma immunoreactive somatomedin C during fasting in humans. J Clin Endocrinol Metab 1981; 53(6):1247–50.

59. Wijngaarden MA, van der Zon GC, van Dijk KW, et al. Effects of prolonged fasting on AMPK signaling, gene expression, and mitochondrial respiratory chain content in skeletal muscle from lean and obese individuals. Am J Physiol Endocrinol Metab 2013;304(9):E1012–21.

60. Grottoli S, Gauna C, Tassone F, et al. Both fasting-induced leptin reduction and GH increase are blunted in Cushing's syndrome and in simple obesity. Clin Endocrinol (Oxf) 2003;58(2):220–8.

61. Pedersen MH, Svart MV, Lebeck J, et al. Substrate metabolism and insulin sensitivity during fasting in obese human subjects: impact of GH blockade. J Clin Endocrinol Metab 2017;102(4):1340–9.

62. Mekala KC, Tritos NA. Effects of recombinant human growth hormone therapy in obesity in adults: a meta analysis. J Clin Endocrinol Metab 2009;94(1):130–7.

63. Bak AM, Moller AB, Vendelbo MH, et al. Differential regulation of lipid and protein metabolism in obese vs. lean subjects before and after a 72-h fast. Am J Physiol Endocrinol Metab 2016;311(1):E224–35.

Effects of Overweight and Obesity in Pregnancy on Health of the Offspring

Margaret L. Dow, MD*, Linda M. Szymanski, MD, PhD

KEYWORDS

- Pregnancy • Offspring • Childhood • Overweight • Obesity

KEY POINTS

- Obesity in pregnancy incurs multiple risks for both the mother and the fetus.
- Many of these risks extend into childhood and even adulthood.
- Congenital, metabolic, allergic/immunologic, cognitive, and behavioral abnormalities occur.
- Optimizing nutrition and exercise in the childbearing years is paramount to interrupting the cycle of obesity.

INTRODUCTION

Obesity is pandemic in the United States and across the globe; according to the most recent statistics, almost two-thirds of adults in the United States are overweight or obese.[1] It affects every aspect of our society: our health, our habits, our work and play, our economy, and even how we socialize. Emerging data support the notion that this is also sadly self-perpetuating. Obesity presents unique concerns for the reproductive-aged woman. Not only does maternal obesity increase pregnancy complications, it also increases the odds of obesity and other metabolic misadventures in offspring, including a panoply of behavioral, cognitive, reproductive, vascular, gastrointestinal, immunologic, and even respiratory derangements. Unfortunately, childhood obesity subsequently tracks into adolescence and adulthood,[2] increasing risk for other chronic diseases, including cardiovascular disease and diabetes.[3]

In this review, we address the link between maternal and childhood obesity. We briefly discuss etiology and outline the potential pregnancy complications that are more common in obese gravidas, followed by the complications that may be experienced in their offspring. We conclude with a discussion of potential lifestyle interventions that may mediate these risks. For purposes of this review, only human subject

Mayo Clinic, 200 First Street Southwest, Rochester, MN 59505, USA
* Corresponding author.
E-mail address: Dow.Margaret@mayo.edu

Endocrinol Metab Clin N Am 49 (2020) 251–263
https://doi.org/10.1016/j.ecl.2020.02.005
0889-8529/20/© 2020 Elsevier Inc. All rights reserved.

studies are presented. When reporting odds ratios (ORs) or hazard ratios (HRs), we present the ratios only, not the confidence interval, for ease of reading.

ETIOLOGY

Many factors, including genetic, biological, behavioral, and environmental, have been implicated as playing a role in the rising epidemic of obesity in children. Although childhood obesity is a multifactorial condition, the link between the maternal and fetal environment appears to play a significant role. The idea that the intrauterine environment, subsequently affecting birthweight, impacted chronic diseases as an adult was initially described in growth-restricted infants[4,5] and has since been extended to large-for-gestational age infants. Studies investigating whether similar mechanisms mediate the metabolic changes induced in utero in situations of undernutrition and overnutrition of the mother appear to suggest that the mechanisms are different; however, more research is needed to understand the metabolic programming, as it is not completely understood.

Twin studies in countries with rigorous birth and health registries have allowed a significant armamentarium of Level IV evidence to help study the determinants of obesity in offspring. As in much of obesity research, the inability to ethically conduct randomized controlled trials limits some of the scientific rigor with which these effects can be studied, particularly in pregnancy and neonates. Murine and other rodent models have elucidated several potential mechanisms mediating childhood obesity. Hypothalamic neural migration,[6] epigenetic changes, and direct endocrine stimulation are just a few of the mechanisms under investigation. The role of epigenetic mechanisms as mediators linking the prenatal environment to changes affecting the offspring's development of obesity is being described in the literature.[7] An example is the elegant analysis that demonstrated methylation sites associated with obesity were significantly higher in offspring of women with obesity than those of normal-weight mothers, a difference not accounted for by gestational weight gain (GWG).[8]

The relationship between the gut microbiome and obesity appears strong, although microbiome changes have not yet been clearly established.[9] Investigating the role of vertical transmission of potentially obesogenic maternal microbiota and neonatal microbiota may augment this pursuit. The microbiome is affected by route of delivery, with numerous studies confirming that cesarean delivery confers a very different and more limited neonatal microbiome than vaginal delivery. Microbiome diversity alone appears to be a sound predictor of adolescent obesity, and this relationship is strengthened by accounting for maternal overweight and obesity.[10] Emerging data support the potential importance of this effect; more than half of the variability in body mass index (BMI) z-scores at age 12 was accounted for by microbiome constituency at age 2, adjusted for delivery mode, exclusive breastfeeding, antibiotic exposure, twins, gestational age at birth, maternal smoking, education, and even after accounting for pre-pregnancy BMI (ppBMI).[11]

Cesarean delivery alone appears to be a risk factor for overweight and obesity in offspring; infant anthropometry shows more rapid growth in the first year of life for infants born by cesarean,[12] and double the risk of obesity at age 20,[13] a difference that persists when accounting for ppBMI, as well as maternal age, education, smoking status, parity, infant birth weight, gestational age, preeclampsia, and gestational diabetes. This interplay of ppBMI and delivery route in affecting childhood obesity appears marked. Compared with offspring born vaginally to women of normal weight, the odds of childhood obesity in offspring of mothers with obesity born by cesarean is almost threefold, just over double for children of cesarean-delivered overweight women, slightly lower for offspring delivered vaginally by obese mothers, and only minimally less for maternal overweight status.[14]

PREGNANCY COMPLICATIONS RESULTING FROM MATERNAL OBESITY

Maternal risks during the pregnancy itself should not be underestimated. A recent meta-analysis estimated 23.9% of all pregnancy complications can be attributed to maternal obesity or overweight.[15] Obese gravidas are more likely to experience a wide variety of pregnancy complications, from difficulty becoming pregnant and increased spontaneous abortions to birth defects, hypertensive disorders, gestational diabetes mellitus (GDM), stillbirth, macrosomia, and even fetal growth restriction. Obese women are much more likely to have an unsuccessful trial of labor and undergo cesarean deliveries. Shoulder dystocia is more frequently experienced by obese women during delivery, possibly resulting in neonatal injury. Erb palsy, a potentially lifelong nerve injury, can result from shoulder dystocia. This risk is increased in infants of mothers with obesity, independent of GDM, at a linear rate of approximately twofold for overweight, almost 2.5-fold for class I obesity, and almost 3.5-fold for class II and above.[16] Ultrasound screening for fetal anomalies may provide suboptimal imaging and, at times, the anatomy screen is unable to be completed. Obese women are also more likely to experience complications from anesthesia (both regional and general). Further complicating the pregnancy and postpartum course for obese women are increased rates of infection and thromboembolism.[17,18] Furthermore, many of the pregnancy complications ultimately result in necessary iatrogenic preterm delivery, exposing the neonate to the additional risks associated with prematurity itself (**Table 1**).

CONGENITAL ANOMALIES

An increased risk of a multitude of birth defects has been attributed to maternal obesity. In the general population, the baseline rate of birth defects is approximately 3%. Aggregate data show that 10 of the more common defects (cleft palate without cleft lip, diaphragmatic hernia, hydrocephalus without spina bifida, hypoplastic left heart syndrome,

---

Table 1
Offspring risks of maternal obesity (body mass index ≥30)

Congenital anomalies	Metabolic abnormalities	Allergy/immunologic issues	Cognition and behavior problems
• Orofacial cleft	• Obesity	• Asthma	• Learning disability
• Septal defects (atrial and ventricular)	• Elevated leptin and other inflammatory markers	• All respiratory hospitalizations	• Attention-deficit disorder
• Hypoplastic left heart	• Insulin resistance	• All-cause pediatric hospitalizations	• Depression
• Transposition of the great vessels	• Diabetes (type 1 and 2)	• Eczema	• Epilepsy
• Tetralogy of Fallot	• Nonalcoholic fatty liver disease	• Leukemia	
• Valve abnormalities	• Early menarche		
• Neural tube defects	• Microbiome shifts		
• Hydrocephaly	• Possible lipid and blood pressure abnormalities		
• Diaphragmatic hernia			
• Omphalocele			
• Cystic kidney			
• Hypospadias			
• Anal atresia,			
• Pes equinovarus			

pulmonary valve atresia and stenosis, pyloric stenosis, rectal and large intestine atresia/stenosis, transposition of great arteries, tetralogy of Fallot, and ventricular septal defects), have a U-shaped relationship with ppBMI, from 3.9% among underweight women to 5.3% among women with class III obesity.[19] In a Swedish study of more than 1 million infants tracked by birth registries, a ppBMI $\geq$40 was associated with a 4.7% prevalence of birth defects, including neural tube defects (OR 4.08), cardiac defects (OR 1.49), and orofacial clefts (OR 1.90). Milder maternal obesity (BMI $\geq$30) has also been associated with a higher risk of congenital anomalies.[20] A prospective cohort study in England supports many of these findings; ppBMI $\geq$30 conferred a statistically significantly increased neonatal risk of ventricular septal defect (adjusted OR 1.56), cleft lip (adjusted OR 3.71), and eye anomalies (adjusted OR 11.36).

When evaluating specific anomalies, *cleft lip and/or palate* has emerged as one of the strongest associations with maternal obesity. A meta-analysis including 8 rigorous studies found an increased risk of all orofacial clefting (OR 1.18) in women with BMIs of 30 or greater.[21] *Cardiac defects* also show a strong association with maternal obesity. A retrospective case-matched study of more than 14,000 infants with heart defects demonstrated increasing OR of maternal obesity by each BMI class, ranging from 1.16 to 1.49. Hypoplastic left heart syndrome and ventricular outflow tract abnormalities were highly associated, as well.[22] *Genital abnormalities*, including hypospadias and cryptorchidism, have shown variable results ranging from no association[23] to an apparent dose-response association between maternal BMI and these malformations.[24]

STILLBIRTH

Stillbirth is clearly associated with maternal obesity. Record-linked cohort analyses show HRs of between 1.51 and 5.7, increasing by obesity class,[16,25] and even more pronounced at late term gestation. Stillbirth risk for women with a BMI of $\geq$50 kg/m^2 was 5.7 times greater than normal-weight women at 39 weeks' gestation, and 13.6 times greater at 41 weeks' gestation.[26] A large cohort analysis of more than 3 million Texas births, including almost 6,000 stillbirths, showed an increase in the overall rate of stillbirth from 15.0 per 10,000 in normal-weight gravidas to 26.7 per 10,000 in morbidly obese gravidas. GDM multiplied the prevalence to 119.9 per 10,000 pregnancies in the normal-weight group and 209.8 per 10,000 pregnancies in the morbidly obese group, a staggering 14-fold difference.[27]

Sadly, a live birth does not preclude *neonatal and infant death*. All-cause neonatal death in offspring of obese mothers is nearly twice as likely, with a V-shaped relationship between BMI and risk of fetal and infant death, lowest at a BMI of 23, independent of anomalies or presence of pregestational diabetes.[28] After adjustment for maternal age at delivery, socioeconomic status, sex of offspring, current age, birth weight, gestation at delivery, and timing of BMI measurement, all-cause mortality remains increased in offspring of obese mothers (BMI >30) compared with mothers with normal BMI (HR 1.35).[29] GWG may also play a role. Studies have suggested a possible U-shaped relationship between GWG and risk of infant death. Bodnar and colleagues[30] controlled for a number of potential confounders and reported that both weight loss and very low weight gain among women with class I-II obesity were associated with high risks of infant mortality. Unfortunately, even with tightly managed GWG, women with obesity remain at higher risk of infant death than those with a normal BMI.

DIABETES

Pre-pregnancy obesity confers some expected and some surprising neonatal and pediatric risks. Long-term studies report an increase in type 2 diabetes mellitus in the offspring of women who are obese and/or diabetic during pregnancy.[31] Collection of umbilical cord blood to evaluate glucose and insulin levels at the time of delivery has revealed evidence of insulin resistance in fetuses of obese women. A strong positive correlation has been noted between maternal and neonatal insulin resistance.[32] This finding of increased insulin resistance with subsequent development of obesity in offspring of obese mothers occurs even when they deliver normal-weight infants.[33] Insulin sensitivity has been shown to be reduced in both early and later childhood. It is unclear whether or not this effect is linear, as different results have been presented and may depend, in part, on maternal ppBMI.[34,35] Metabolic syndrome risk is also increased, even in the first decade of life.[36] Risk of type 1 diabetes follows interesting patterns: offspring risk is increased with either parent having type 1 diabetes, regardless of BMI, and also appears to be increased by approximately one-third in offspring of obese mothers even if *neither* parent has underlying diabetes.[37]

CARDIOMETABOLIC EFFECTS

Cardiometabolic outcomes have proven difficult to parse out. Although some evidence shows no increase in markers for poor cardiometabolic outcomes after correcting for BMI, including increased blood pressure, elevated triglycerides, low high-density lipoprotein (HDL), and high sensitivity C-reactive protein (hs-CRP),[38] Leibowitz and colleagues[39] identified an almost 16-fold increase in hs-CRP, without elevations in other inflammatory markers (tumor necrosis factor-alpha, interleukin-6, and adiponectin) in the offspring with obese mothers compared with those without. Using a combined metabolic profile, (waist-to-hip ratio, systolic blood pressure, diastolic blood pressure, fasting glucose, triglycerides, and HDL-cholesterol), Oostvogels and colleagues[40] identified a clear association between increased risk and ppBMI, not weakened by accounting for neonatal weight. Similarly, early findings of a longitudinal multigeneration study of Australian women and their offspring using genetic, serum, sociologic, environmental, familial, and psychological markers of disease reported associations among maternal obesity, early mid-GWG, and socioeconomic status with nonalcoholic fatty liver disease (NAFLD), adiposity, and cardiometabolic dysfunction in offspring.[41]

NONALCOHOLIC FATTY LIVER DISEASE

Multiple studies identified a relationship between parental obesity and NAFLD. Increased neonatal fat deposition in the liver is present in offspring of mothers with obesity,[42,43] and is more marked in mothers with obesity and GDM.[44] Interestingly, there may be a gender effect, with maternal ppBMI and higher weight gain before 18 weeks (defined as $\geq$6 kg) conferring increased risk of NAFLD in female offspring. NAFLD in male offspring was associated with higher paternal BMI, maternal ppBMI, and lower socioeconomic status, although parental BMI associations attenuated with consideration of other offspring metabolic factors.[45]

OVERALL HOSPITALIZATIONS

Evaluating all-cause hospitalization in an Australian cohort of children younger than 6 born to mothers with obesity demonstrates almost 50% higher rates of admission, most pronounced for diagnoses of conditions of the nervous system, infections, metabolic conditions, perinatal conditions, injuries, and respiratory conditions, with relative risks (RRs) ranging from 1.3 to 4.0.[46] A Scottish study using record-linked cohort analysis shows a specific increased risk of hospital admission for a cardiovascular event (HR 1.29) in these offspring.[29]

EMOTIONAL AND BEHAVIORAL HEALTH

Maternal obesity confers a higher risk of attention-deficit/hyperactivity disorder (ADHD) and autism spectrum disorders (ASDs) in the offspring. A large Danish birth cohort analyzed these associations and found that compared with normal-weight mothers, the risk of having a child with ADHD was increased in overweight women (HR 1.28), more so in women with obesity (HR 1.47), and even more in women with severe obesity (HR 1.95). The same pattern was seen for the combined ADHD and ASD group. The risk for ASDs alone was increased by maternal underweight status (HR 1.30) and maternal obesity (HR 1.39).[47] A deeper analysis of self-control behaviors related to ADHD also identified an association with increasing maternal ppBMI,[48] while executive function and tolerance of delayed gratification was decreased in children of women with class III obesity.[49] A dual-population study showed total behavior problems appeared increased in offspring of women with overweight in one subgroup but not the other, although associations of child attention problems, emotional problems, or nonverbal skills were inconsistent and nonsignificant.[50] Another study using the Behavior Problems Index (BPI) identified a gender difference in maternal effects, with boys ages 9 to 11 with mothers with obesity class II or greater showing significantly higher BPI score.[51]

Early work investigated the association of offspring schizophrenia and maternal ppBMI; however, results are conflicting. Jones and colleagues[52] found no effect, whereas the combination of maternal age, parity, and ppBMI appeared to confer higher risk in another study.[53] This relationship may be affected by other factors over time. A study evaluating adult offspring in 1959 to 1965 found a relative risk of developing a schizophrenia spectrum disorder of 2.9, independent of maternal age, parity, race, education, or cigarette smoking during pregnancy.[54] Maternal obesity also has been implicated in the development of childhood eating disorders, maternal body dissatisfaction, internalization of the "thin-ideal," dieting, and bulimic symptoms, and both maternal and paternal BMI appear to prospectively predict the emergence of childhood eating disturbances,[55] although these relationships may merit further dissecting.

LOWER IQ

A study of 2 Finnish populations, 20 years apart, showed emergence of a new association of formally diagnosed intellectual disability in offspring of mothers with ppBMI ≥30 in the latter group that did not appear in the former (adjusted OR 2.8).[56] This association is inconsistent in later works that identified no significant differences in cognitive function between offspring of normal maternal ppBMI and those with maternal obesity when controlled for confounders.[50,57]

CEREBRAL PALSY

Several individual studies demonstrate a clear relationship between maternal obesity and cerebral palsy (CP), and studies that analyzed results by class of obesity show a linear relationship between relative risk of CP and increasing obesity.[58–60] A small increase in risk has even been reported with overweight status,[61] although another study, stratified by gestational age and magnesium exposure (a neuroprotectant in preterm infants) was less compelling.[62] Obstetrically, it is well established that preterm birth is an independent risk factor for CP, which may complicate this area of research. However, a meta-analysis, which includes the McPherson study, showed a relationship. Looking at more than 12,000 cases, pooled ORs for CP in offspring according to maternal obesity were 1.31 for class I, 1.65 for class II, and 2.37 for class III obesity.[63] An additional small study looked at both CP and epilepsy risk by maternal ppBMI, supporting the association of the former but not the latter.[59]

EPILEPSY

Although neonatal seizures may be part of the CP spectrum, additional studies have looked at childhood epilepsy alone. Analyzing a cohort of more than 1.4 million births in Sweden, hazard risks of epilepsy by maternal BMI categories were 1.11 for maternal overweight, 1.20 for class I obesity, 1.30 for class II, and nearly double, 1.82, for mothers with class III obesity. These findings were adjusted for a number of maternal and neonatal confounders with not only persistence of the effect of maternal obesity but also a compounding of overall risk.

ASTHMA, ECZEMA, AND ALLERGY

Although markers of inflammation are a current area of much inquiry, the relationship between childhood atopy and maternal obesity is well supported by many studies. The risk of hospitalization for respiratory illness before age 5 appears to increase from minimal additional risk for offspring of overweight mothers (OR 1.08) to 1.29 for obese mothers.[64] In a large Danish study, childhood asthma/wheezing but not atopic eczema or hayfever during the first 7 years of life was partly explained by increases in ppBMI, and to a lesser extent by excess GWG.[65] Other studies have shown the relationship between maternal BMI and asthma to extend to offspring up to the age of 16 when the mother was in the obese, but not overweight, category.[66] Their results also suggested that the offspring's BMI may partly mediate the relationship. There may be gender differences here, as well, although the data are unclear.[67,68]

CANCER

Limited studies suggest a relationship between maternal overweight/obesity and cancer in the offspring. A retrospective analysis looking at childhood cancers in aggregate suggests maternal overweight status appears to be associated with higher risk of childhood leukemias other than acute myeloid leukemia and acute lymphocytic leukemia, with excessive GWG incurring higher risk for astrocytomas.[69] These findings are further substantiated by a recent study showing a 57% higher leukemia risk by age 14 in children born to mothers with class III obesity; large newborn size was associated with a greater than twofold risk of any cancer, which did not mitigate the effects of maternal obesity alone.[70]

EARLY PUBERTY

Early menarche is associated with multiple adverse health outcomes in adulthood. Its association with ppBMI appears significant even with maternal overweight status, and even after controlling for birth weight, prepubertal BMI, and maternal GWG.[71] This is somewhat divergent from earlier findings. A 2009 analysis showed an increased risk of menarche before age 12 in offspring of mothers with ppBMI ≥30, OR 3.3, although not with overweight status,[72] whereas another prospective longitudinal study showed attenuation of this effect when accounting for prepubertal BMI in offspring.[73] Looking more broadly at thelarche (breast development) and pubarche (development of pubic hair), a recent US study supported the role of both maternal obesity and excess GWG, HR 2.0, slightly diminished but still significant after adjusting for girls' prepubertal BMI.[74]

INTERVENTIONS TO REDUCE CHILDHOOD OBESITY

As outlined previously, research clearly shows that maternal obesity and related issues may have a wide range of adverse effects on the health of the offspring, which then have long-term consequences. Thus, pregnancy provides an opportunity to intervene with lifestyle modifications that may benefit maternal health, leading to improved pregnancy outcomes and possible health benefits for the offspring. Ideally, achieving a healthy weight before pregnancy would be the most effective way to improve obstetric outcomes; however, data trends indicate that the percentage of obese pregnant women is increasing. In nonpregnant individuals, evidence strongly supports that adherence to a healthy lifestyle reduces risk of morbidity and mortality in women.[75–77] Similarly, physical activity provides significant benefits for pregnant women, including a reduction in the risk of developing GDM and reducing GWG.[78] These 2 changes may lead to improved metabolic parameters in pregnant women, which may then be transferred to the offspring. Meta-analysis on GDM risk reduction with exercise shows that the greatest magnitude in risk reduction is seen when the exercise is started pre-pregnancy, resulting in a 55% reduction in risk in most active compared with the least active women. When exercise was started in early pregnancy, a 24% reduction in GDM was seen.[79] It has also been shown that physically active pregnant women gain less weight than inactive women and are less likely to exceed the Institute of Medicine's weight gain recommendations.[80] This in turn lowers their risk of excessive postpartum weight retention, future obesity, and birth of an infant with macrosomia.[81]

Prospective data looking at the impact of a variety of healthy lifestyle practices on obesity in the offspring suggest that pregnant women who adhere to these behaviors, including healthy eating, healthy BMI, abstinence from smoking, and increased physical activity, have a significantly lower risk of their offspring developing obesity.[82] Studies that have attempted to prospectively evaluate the effects of exercise interventions (or diet plus exercise) in obese women on maternal and/or neonatal outcomes report conflicting results.[18,83–86] However, methodological differences, including exercise routines and different follow-up protocols, may account for these differences. The bottom line is that data are quite clear regarding the health benefits of regular physical activity for adults and children,[81] and it would be difficult to imagine that appropriately prescribed physical activity would not be beneficial during pregnancy in these high-risk women, for both the woman and her offspring. Pregnancy provides an ideal opportunity for women to attempt to improve not only their own health, in the short and long term, but also the health of their offspring before they are even born.

SUMMARY

Maternal obesity clearly confers a host of potential pregnancy complications as well as adverse health effects on offspring. Ironically, though, much of this research may be dismissed prematurely. In efforts to account for lifestyle factors, many of the studies adjust results for offspring BMI, weight, and/or adiposity, and the statistical significance seems to disappear. The desire to mete out in utero effects versus early life exposures is admirable and stimulates our scientific minds. Is the cycle of obesity secondary to nature or nurture? The answer is yes: both. Efforts to control for maternal BMI, paternal BMI, adolescent BMI, diabetes, adiposity, and many other factors may help identify targets for intervention, but this must not overshadow efforts at both primary prevention and early intervention. Aggressive but realistic preconceptual diet, physical activity, and other lifestyle changes may help optimize maternal health, leading to an improvement in the in utero environment, and ultimately effecting changes in the health of the offspring. Perhaps these maternal and offspring health improvements can help break this cycle.

DISCLOSURE

The authors have nothing to disclose.

REFERENCES

1. Hales CM, Carroll MD, Fryar CD, et al. Prevalence of obesity among adults and youth: United States, 2015-2016. NCHS Data Brief 2017;288:1–8.
2. Freedman DS, Lawman HG, Galuska DA, et al. Tracking and variability in childhood levels of BMI: The Bogalusa Heart Study. Obesity (Silver Spring) 2018; 26(7):1197–202.
3. Raitakari OT, Juonala M, Kähönen M, et al. Cardiovascular risk factors in childhood and carotid artery intima-media thickness in adulthood: the Cardiovascular Risk in Young Finns Study. JAMA 2003;290(17):2277–83.
4. Barker DJ, Bull AR, Osmond C, et al. Fetal and placental size and risk of hypertension in adult life. BMJ 1990;301(6746):259–62.
5. Hales CN, Barker DJ. The thrifty phenotype hypothesis. Br Med Bull 2001; 60:5–20.
6. Stachowiak EK, Oommen S, Vasu VT, et al. Maternal obesity affects gene expression and cellular development in fetal brains. Nutr Neurosci 2013;16(3):96–103.
7. Desai M, Jellyman JK, Ross MG. Epigenomics, gestational programming and risk of metabolic syndrome. Int J Obes (Lond) 2015;39(4):633–41.
8. Sharp GC, Lawlor DA, Richmond RC, et al. Maternal pre-pregnancy BMI and gestational weight gain, offspring DNA methylation and later offspring adiposity: findings from the Avon Longitudinal Study of Parents and Children. Int J Epidemiol 2015;44(4):1288–304.
9. Maruvada P, Leone V, Kaplan LM, et al. The human microbiome and obesity: moving beyond associations. Cell Host Microbe 2017;22(5):589–99.
10. Tun HM, Bridgman SL, Chari R, et al. Roles of birth mode and infant gut microbiota in intergenerational transmission of overweight and obesity from mother to offspring. JAMA Pediatr 2018;172(4):368–77.
11. Stanislawski MA, Dabelea D, Wagner BD, et al. Gut microbiota in the first 2 years of life and the association with body mass index at age 12 in a Norwegian birth cohort. MBio 2018;9(5) [pii:e01751-18].
12. Mueller NT, Zhang M, Hoyo C, et al. Does cesarean delivery impact infant weight gain and adiposity over the first year of life? Int J Obes (Lond) 2019;43(8): 1549–55.
13. Hansen S, Halldorsson TI, Olsen SF, et al. Birth by cesarean section in relation to adult offspring overweight and biomarkers of cardiometabolic risk. Int J Obes (Lond) 2018;42(1):15–9.
14. Mueller NT, Mao G, Bennet WL, et al. Does vaginal delivery mitigate or strengthen the intergenerational association of overweight and obesity? Findings from the Boston Birth Cohort. Int J Obes (Lond) 2017;41(4):497–501.
15. Santos S, Voerman E, Amiano P, et al. Impact of maternal body mass index and gestational weight gain on pregnancy complications: an individual participant data meta-analysis of European, North American and Australian cohorts. BJOG 2019;126(8):984–95.

16. Hilden K, Hanson U, Persson M, et al. Gestational diabetes and adiposity are independent risk factors for perinatal outcomes: a population based cohort study in Sweden. Diabet Med 2019;36(2):151–7.

17. ACOG Practice Bulletin No 156: Obesity in pregnancy. Obstet Gynecol 2015; 126(6):e112–26.

18. Seneviratne SN, McCowan LM, Cutfield WS, et al. Exercise in pregnancies complicated by obesity: achieving benefits and overcoming barriers. Am J Obstet Gynecol 2015;212(4):442–9.

19. Block SR, Watkins SM, Salemi JL, et al. Maternal pre-pregnancy body mass index and risk of selected birth defects: evidence of a dose-response relationship. Paediatr Perinat Epidemiol 2013;27(6):521–31.

20. Blomberg MI, Kallen B. Maternal obesity and morbid obesity: the risk for birth defects in the offspring. Birth Defects Res 2010;88(1):35–40.

21. Blanco R, Colombo A, Suazo J. Maternal obesity is a risk factor for orofacial clefts: a meta-analysis. Br J Oral Maxillofac Surg 2015;53(8):699–704.

22. Madsen NL, Schwartz SM, Lewin MB, et al. Prepregnancy body mass index and congenital heart defects among offspring: a population-based study. Congenit Heart Dis 2013;8(2):131–41.

23. Adams SV, Hastert TA, Huang Y, et al. No association between maternal pre-pregnancy obesity and risk of hypospadias or cryptorchidism in male newborns. Birth Defects Res A Clin Mol Teratol 2011;91(4):241–8.

24. Arendt LH, Ramlau-Hansen CH, Lindhard MS, et al. Maternal overweight and obesity and genital anomalies in male offspring: a population-based Swedish cohort study. Paediatr Perinat Epidemiol 2017;31(4):317–27.

25. Vasudevan C, Renfrew M, McGuire W. Fetal and perinatal consequences of maternal obesity. Arch Dis Child Fetal Neonatal Ed 2011;96(5):F378–82.

26. Yao R, Ananth CV, Park BY, et al, Perinatal Research Consortium. Obesity and the risk of stillbirth: a population-based cohort study. Am J Obstet Gynecol 2014; 210(5):457.e1-9.

27. Browne K, Park BY, Goetzinger KR, et al. The joint effects of obesity and pregestational diabetes on the risk of stillbirth. J Matern Fetal Neonatal Med 2019;1–7.

28. Tennant PW, Rankin J, Bell R. Maternal body mass index and the risk of fetal and infant death: a cohort study from the North of England. Hum Reprod 2011;26(6): 1501–11.

29. Reynolds RM, Allan KM, Raja EA, et al. Maternal obesity during pregnancy and premature mortality from cardiovascular event in adult offspring: follow-up of 1 323 275 person years. BMJ 2013;347:f4539.

30. Bodnar LM, Siminerio LL, Himes KP, et al. Maternal obesity and gestational weight gain are risk factors for infant death. Obesity (Silver Spring) 2016;24(2): 490–8.

31. Dabelea D, Pettitt DJ. Intrauterine diabetic environment confers risks for type 2 diabetes mellitus and obesity in the offspring, in addition to genetic susceptibility. J Pediatr Endocrinol Metab 2001;14(8):1085–91.

32. Catalano PM, Farrell K, Thomas A, et al. Perinatal risk factors for childhood obesity and metabolic dysregulation. Am J Clin Nutr 2009;90(5):1303–13.

33. Mingrone G, Manco M, Mora ME, et al. Influence of maternal obesity on insulin sensitivity and secretion in offspring. Diabetes Care 2008;31(9):1872–6.

34. Maftei O, Whitrow MJ, Davies MJ, et al. Maternal body size prior to pregnancy, gestational diabetes and weight gain: associations with insulin resistance in children at 9-10 years. Diabet Med 2015;32(2):174–80.

35. Derraik JG, Ayyavoo A, Hofman PL, et al. Increasing maternal prepregnancy body mass index is associated with reduced insulin sensitivity and increased blood pressure in their children. Clin Endocrinol 2015;83(3):352–6.
36. Boney CM, Verma A, Tucker R, et al. Metabolic syndrome in childhood: association with birth weight, maternal obesity, and gestational diabetes mellitus. Pediatrics 2005;115(3):e290–6.
37. Hussen HI, Persson M, Moradi T. Maternal overweight and obesity are associated with increased risk of type 1 diabetes in offspring of parents without diabetes regardless of ethnicity. Diabetologia 2015;58(7):1464–73.
38. Gaillard R, Welten M, Oddy WH, et al. Associations of maternal prepregnancy body mass index and gestational weight gain with cardio-metabolic risk factors in adolescent offspring: a prospective cohort study. BJOG 2016;123(2):207–16.
39. Leibowitz KL, Moore RH, Ahima RS, et al. Maternal obesity associated with inflammation in their children. World J Pediatr 2012;8(1):76–9.
40. Oostvogels AJ, Stronks K, Roseboom TJ, et al. Maternal prepregnancy BMI, offspring's early postnatal growth, and metabolic profile at age 5-6 years: the ABCD Study. J Clin Endocrinol Metab 2014;99(10):3845–54.
41. Dontje ML, Eastwood P, Straker L. Western Australian pregnancy cohort (Raine) Study: generation 1. BMJ Open 2019;9(5):e026276.
42. Santos S, Monnereau C, Felix JF, et al. Maternal body mass index, gestational weight gain, and childhood abdominal, pericardial, and liver fat assessed by magnetic resonance imaging. Int J Obes (Lond) 2019;43(3):581–93.
43. Ayonrinde OT, Oddy WH, Adams LA, et al. Infant nutrition and maternal obesity influence the risk of non-alcoholic fatty liver disease in adolescents. J Hepatol 2017;67(3):568–76.
44. Brumbaugh DE, Tearse P, Cree-Green M, et al. Intrahepatic fat is increased in the neonatal offspring of obese women with gestational diabetes. J Pediatr 2013; 162(5):930–6.e1.
45. Ayonrinde OT, Adams LA, Mori TA, et al. Sex differences between parental pregnancy characteristics and nonalcoholic fatty liver disease in adolescents. Hepatology 2018;67(1):108–22.
46. Cameron CM, Shibl R, McClure RJ, et al. Maternal pregravid body mass index and child hospital admissions in the first 5 years of life: results from an Australian birth cohort. Int J Obes 2014;38(10):1268–74.
47. Andersen CH, Thomsen PH, Nohr EA, et al. Maternal body mass index before pregnancy as a risk factor for ADHD and autism in children. Eur Child Adolesc Psychiatry 2018;27(2):139–48.
48. Fuemmeler BF, Zucker N, Sheng Y, et al. Pre-pregnancy weight and symptoms of attention deficit hyperactivity disorder and executive functioning behaviors in preschool children. Int J Environ Res Public Health 2019;16(4) [pii:E667].
49. Mina TH, Lahti M, Drake AJ, et al. Prenatal exposure to maternal very severe obesity is associated with impaired neurodevelopment and executive functioning in children. Pediatr Res 2017;82(1):47–54.
50. Brion MJ, Zeegers M, Jaddoe V, et al. Intrauterine effects of maternal prepregnancy overweight on child cognition and behavior in 2 cohorts. Pediatrics 2011;127(1):e202–11.
51. Deardorff J, Smith LH, Petito L, et al. Maternal prepregnancy weight and children's behavioral and emotional outcomes. Am J Prev Med 2017;53(4):432–40.
52. Jones PB, Rantakallio P, Hartikainen AL, et al. Schizophrenia as a long-term outcome of pregnancy, delivery, and perinatal complications: a 28-year follow-

up of the 1966 north Finland general population birth cohort. Am J Psychiatry 1998;155(3):355–64.

53. Kawai M, Minabe Y, Takagai S, et al. Poor maternal care and high maternal body mass index in pregnancy as a risk factor for schizophrenia in offspring. Acta Psychiatr Scand 2004;110(4):257–63.

54. Schaefer CA, Brown AS, Wyatt RJ, et al. Maternal prepregnant body mass and risk of schizophrenia in adult offspring. Schizophr Bull 2000;26(2):275–86.

55. Stice E, Agras WS, Hammer LD. Risk factors for the emergence of childhood eating disturbances: a five-year prospective study. Int J Eat Disord 1999;25(4):375–87.

56. Heikura U, Taanila A, Hartikainen AL, et al. Variations in prenatal sociodemographic factors associated with intellectual disability: a study of the 20-year interval between two birth cohorts in northern Finland. Am J Epidemiol 2008;167(2):169–77.

57. Bliddal M, Olsen J, Stovring H, et al. Maternal pre-pregnancy BMI and intelligence quotient (IQ) in 5-year-old children: a cohort based study. PLoS One 2014;9(4):e94498.

58. Crisham Janik MD, Newman TB, Cheng YW, et al. Maternal diagnosis of obesity and risk of cerebral palsy in the child. J Pediatr 2013;163(5):1307–12.

59. Pan C, Deroche CB, Mann JR, et al. Is prepregnancy obesity associated with risk of cerebral palsy and epilepsy in children? J Child Neurol 2014;29(12):NP196–201.

60. Forthun I, Wilcox AJ, Strandberg-Larsen K, et al. Maternal prepregnancy BMI and risk of cerebral palsy in offspring. Pediatrics 2016;138(4) [pii:e20160874].

61. Villamor E, Tedroff K, Peterson M, et al. Association between maternal body mass index in early pregnancy and incidence of cerebral palsy. JAMA 2017;317(9):925–36.

62. McPherson JA, Smid MC, Smiley S, et al. Association of maternal obesity with child cerebral palsy or death. Am J Perinatol 2017;34(6):563–7.

63. Zhang J, Peng L, Chang Q, et al. Maternal obesity and risk of cerebral palsy in children: a systematic review and meta-analysis. Dev Med Child Neurol 2019;61(1):31–8.

64. Parsons EC, Patel K, Tran BT, et al. Maternal pre-gravid obesity and early childhood respiratory hospitalization: a population-based case-control study. Matern Child Health J 2013;17(6):1095–102.

65. Harpsoe MC, Basit S, Bager P, et al. Maternal obesity, gestational weight gain, and risk of asthma and atopic disease in offspring: a study within the Danish National Birth Cohort. J Allergy Clin Immunol 2013;131(4):1033–40.

66. Ekstrom S, Magnusson J, Kull I, et al. Maternal body mass index in early pregnancy and offspring asthma, rhinitis and eczema up to 16 years of age. Clin Exp Allergy 2015;45(1):283–91.

67. Quek YW, Sun HL, Ng YY, et al. Associations of serum leptin with atopic asthma and allergic rhinitis in children. Am J Rhinol Allergy 2010;24(5):354–8.

68. Guler N, Kirerleri E, Ones U, et al. Leptin: does it have any role in childhood asthma? J Allergy Clin Immunol 2004;114(2):254–9.

69. Contreras ZA, Ritz B, Virk J, et al. Maternal pre-pregnancy and gestational diabetes, obesity, gestational weight gain, and risk of cancer in young children: a population-based study in California. Cancer Causes Control 2016;27(10):1273–85.

70. Stacy SL, Buchanich JM, Ma ZQ, et al. Maternal obesity, birth size, and risk of childhood cancer development. Am J Epidemiol 2019;188(8):1503–11.

71. Deardorff J, Berry-Millett R, Rehkopf D, et al. Maternal pre-pregnancy BMI, gestational weight gain, and age at menarche in daughters. Matern Child Health J 2013;17(8):1391–8.
72. Keim SA, Branum AM, Klebanoff MA, et al. Maternal body mass index and daughters' age at menarche. Epidemiology 2009;20(5):677–81.
73. Lawn RB, Lawlor DA, Fraser A. Associations between maternal prepregnancy body mass index and gestational weight gain and daughter's age at menarche: the Avon Longitudinal Study of parents and children. Am J Epidemiol 2018; 187(4):677–86.
74. Aghaee S, Laurent CA, Deardorff J, et al. Associations of maternal gestational weight gain and obesity with the timing of pubertal onset in daughters. Am J Epidemiol 2019;188(7):1262–9.
75. Stampfer MJ, Hu FB, Manson JE, et al. Primary prevention of coronary heart disease in women through diet and lifestyle. N Engl J Med 2000;343(1):16–22.
76. Hu FB, Manson JE, Stampfer MJ, et al. Diet, lifestyle, and the risk of type 2 diabetes mellitus in women. N Engl J Med 2001;345(11):790–7.
77. van Dam RM, Li T, Spiegelman D, et al. Combined impact of lifestyle factors on mortality: prospective cohort study in US women. BMJ 2008;337:a1440.
78. ACOG Committee Opinion No. 650: Physical activity and exercise during pregnancy and the postpartum period. Obstet Gynecol 2015;126(6):e135–42.
79. Tobias DK, Zhang C, van Dam RM, et al. Physical activity before and during pregnancy and risk of gestational diabetes mellitus: a meta-analysis. Diabetes Care 2011;34(1):223–9.
80. Streuling I, Beyerlein A, Rosenfeld E, et al. Physical activity and gestational weight gain: a meta-analysis of intervention trials. BJOG 2011;118(3):278–84.
81. DiPietro L, Buchner DM, Marquez DX, et al. New scientific basis for the 2018 U.S. physical activity guidelines. J Sport Health Sci 2019;8(3):197–200.
82. Dhana K, Haines J, Liu G, et al. Association between maternal adherence to healthy lifestyle practices and risk of obesity in offspring: results from two prospective cohort studies of mother-child pairs in the United States. BMJ 2018; 362:k2486.
83. Tanvig M. Offspring body size and metabolic profile - effects of lifestyle intervention in obese pregnant women. Dan Med J 2014;61(7):B4893.
84. Grivell RM, O'Brien CM, Dodd JM. Managing obesity in pregnancy: a change in focus from harm minimization to prevention. Semin Reprod Med 2016;34(2): e38–46.
85. Wang C, Wei Y, Zhang X, et al. A randomized clinical trial of exercise during pregnancy to prevent gestational diabetes mellitus and improve pregnancy outcome in overweight and obese pregnant women. Am J Obstet Gynecol 2017;216(4): 340–51.
86. Poston L. Do physical activity interventions prevent gestational diabetes? BJOG 2015;122(9):1175.

Iatrogenic Obesity

Rekha B. Kumar, MD, MS, DABOM*, Louis J. Aronne, MD, DABOM

KEYWORDS

- Medication-induced obesity • Medication-induced weight gain
- Weight profile of antipsychotic medications
- Weight-centric approach of diabetes management

KEY POINTS

- Commonly prescribed medicines may cause weight gain.
- Most common agents known to do this are antipsychotics, antidepressants, and antiepileptics, insulin, insulin secretagogues, and antihypertensive medicines.
- When treating medication-induced weight gain, medications should not be changed or adjusted without consulting with the initial prescriber, and the important of a calorie-restricted diet and increased physical activity to treat the obesity should be emphasized.

INTRODUCTION

Several commonly prescribed medicines can contribute to abnormal weight gain or interfere with patients' ability to lose weight. Physicians should be able to identify these medications and consider substituting with medicines that are weight neutral, or agents that can treat the underlying condition and cause weight loss at the same time if that change is appropriate. Use of over-the-counter medications and supplements should be reviewed in order to identify factors contributing to weight gain. Not all medicines affect patients' weight the same way; although some cause weight gain in one patient, they may induce weight loss in another. Others may lead to weight loss initially but cause weight gain when taken long term. Often, a drug's effect on a patient's weight depends on the patient's medical history and lifestyle, including factors such as baseline glucose tolerance, diet, and exercise level.

Commonly prescribed medicines that may cause weight gain include antipsychotics, antidepressants, and antiepileptics. In diabetes treatment, insulin and insulin secretagogues can further compound the obesity problem that led to diabetes to begin with, thus creating a vicious cycle. There are antihypertensives with weight gain–promoting properties that can be substituted with many other weight-neutral options. In addition, glucocorticoids, progestational hormones and

Weill Cornell Medicine, Comprehensive Weight Control Center, 1165 York Avenue, New York, NY 10065, USA
* Corresponding author. Division of Endocrinology, Diabetes, and Metabolism, Weill Cornell Medicine, Comprehensive Weight Control Center, 1165 York Avenue, New York, NY 10065.
E-mail address: Reb9037@med.cornell.edu
Twitter: @DrRekhaKumar (R.B.K.)

Endocrinol Metab Clin N Am 49 (2020) 265–273
https://doi.org/10.1016/j.ecl.2020.02.010
0889-8529/20/© 2020 Elsevier Inc. All rights reserved.

implants, antihistamines, and oral contraceptives may contribute to weight gain in certain patients.[1]

ANTIDEPRESSANTS AND ANTIPSYCHOTICS

For patients with psychiatric conditions, weight gain is a common complaint and often multifactorial. Individuals with psychiatric illnesses are at an increased risk of developing metabolic derangements because of multiple factors, including the medications they require for treatment. The antidepressant medications used for treatment frequently contribute to weight gain and/or make weight loss more difficult to achieve. Among the numerous antidepressants, there is a broad range of weight gain potential, typically influenced by the duration of therapy.[2] Early weight gain after initiation of therapy is a strong predictor of long-term weight change.

Within the selective serotonin reuptake inhibitor (SSRI) and tricyclic antidepressant (TCA) classes of drugs, paroxetine and amitriptyline respectively are associated with the greatest risk for weight gain.[3,4] Lithium, mirtazapine, and the monoamine oxidase inhibitors (MAOIs) are also associated with weight gain.[5] There are only a limited number of antidepressants that are not associated with weight gain. The SSRIs fluoxetine and sertraline have been associated with weight loss with short-term use and relative weight neutrality with long-term use.[5,6] In a meta-analysis of 116 studies, SSRIs, including fluoxetine and sertraline, were found to be associated with weight loss in short-term use (4–12 weeks) and weight neutrality in long-term use (>4 months).[4] In patients with type 2 diabetes, fluoxetine was associated with weight loss of 5.1 kg (range, 3.3–6.9 kg) at 24 to 26 weeks' follow-up.[6] No significant weight effect was observed for citalopram or escitalopram; however, the effect of each antidepressant may vary greatly depending on an individual's characteristics.[4]

In a systematic review and meta-analysis of 257 randomized trials, weight gain was associated with the use of amitriptyline (1.8 kg) and mirtazapine (1.5 kg), whereas weight loss was associated with the use of bupropion (1.3 kg) and fluoxetine (1.3 kg). Bupropion is the only antidepressant that has been shown to consistently promote weight loss.[5] Bupropion is a norepinephrine and dopamine reuptake inhibitor approved for the treatment of depression and to assist with smoking cessation. Bupropion has been shown to decrease body weight by suppressing appetite and reducing food cravings.[7,8] It was approved by the US Food and Drug Administration (FDA) for chronic weight management in 2014 in combination with another medication, naltrexone, under the brand name Contrave. Depending on the nature of the patient's depression, bupropion, fluoxetine, or sertraline might be reasonable alternatives to prevent or reduce weight gain in patients requiring antidepressant medication.

Because different classes of antidepressants are typically prescribed for different types of depression, the few agents that are weight neutral and weight loss promoting are not appropriate for all patients with depression. For example, bupropion can be activating, so it could potentially exacerbate anxiety or be inappropriate for patients with bipolar disorder. Thus, patients with concomitant depression and anxiety might be better candidates for a different antidepressant, which could lead to some weight gain but would better manage the individuals' symptoms. In such cases, it is prudent to prescribe the lowest dose required for clinical efficacy for the shortest duration necessary. Significant early weight gain should prompt physicians to consider other therapeutic options and/or to initiate additional weight-controlling strategies. The choice of antidepressant must ultimately be guided by best practice for the individual patient's circumstance.[9]

With respect to the antipsychotics, there are few weight-neutral options. Olanzapine, clozapine, quetiapine, and risperidone are consistently associated with weight gain,[10,11] and studies show that patients may lose weight and develop improved glucose tolerance when switched from olanzapine to ziprasidone.[12] Even the options that seem weight neutral in short clinical trials show substantial variability in terms of each patient's individual weight change, especially with longer-term use. Lurasidone and ziprasidone seem to be the most weight neutral in the class, with aripiprazole generally showing a lower risk for weight gain as well.[13] The antipsychotics seem to affect weight via multiple mechanisms, including effects on central appetite, satiety, and energy homeostasis pathways via alterations of dopaminergic, serotonergic, and histaminergic neurotransmission.[14–16] Additional effects on endocannabinoid receptors, several neuropeptides, hormones, and cytokines seem to play a role.[16]

It is rarely possible to replace the mood-stabilizing effects of an antipsychotic medication with a different class of medication. However, combining an antipsychotic with another class of medication can often help to reduce the dose of antipsychotic required for treatment. Antiepileptics are frequently combined with antipsychotics in this manner. Antiepileptic agents have broad-ranging effects on weight, with some associated with substantial weight gain and others promoting weight loss. Valproic acid, gabapentin, pregabalin, and carbamazepine are associated with weight gain, whereas lamotrigine, levetiracetam, and phenytoin are considered relatively weight neutral.[17,18] Topiramate and zonisamide have been consistently associated with weight loss.[19] In addition to antiseizure activity, a subset of the antiepileptics are used off label to treat psychiatric conditions, specifically bipolar disorder. Topiramate monotherapy is FDA approved for both the treatment of migraines and the management of seizures, and is used off label as a mood stabilizer in patients with bipolar disorder.

Metformin is typically the first-line agent to mitigate weight gain associated with antipsychotic medication use.[20] Metformin is FDA approved for the treatment of type 2 diabetes mellitus (T2DM) but is commonly used off label for other conditions, including T2DM prevention in patients with prediabetes or impaired fasting glucose, treatment of polycystic ovarian syndrome, and obesity/overweight, especially in patients with drug-induced weight gain.[21] In addition to metformin, off-label topiramate can be used to facilitate weight loss in antipsychotic-induced weight gain. Topiramate was approved by the FDA for chronic weight management in 2012 in combination with another medication, phentermine, under the brand name Qsymia.

When possible, practitioners should use weight-neutral or weight loss–promoting medications in the treatment of psychiatric conditions. If this is not feasible, weight gain can be prevented or lessened by selecting the lowest dose required to produce clinical efficacy for the shortest duration necessary. The addition of dedicated anti-obesity medications (liraglutide 3.0 mg [Saxenda], phentermine/topiramate extended release [ER] [Qymia], lorcaserin [Belviq], or naltrexone/bupropion ER [Contrave]) could be considered on a case-by-case basis, as directed by an obesity medicine specialist. Lifestyle modification, including diet and exercise counseling, is the cornerstone of treatment of obesity management and should be encouraged in tandem with all pharmacologic treatment approaches, especially when a patient requires medication that can cause weight gain. **Table 1** presents an overview of the weight profiles of several antidepressant and antipsychotic medications.[13]

ANTIHYPERTENSIVES

β-Adrenergic blockers have been shown to promote weight gain and inhibit weight loss, especially in patients with hypertension and diabetes.[22] In addition to potential

Table 1
Psychiatric medications associated with weight gain, weight neutrality, and weight loss

	Weight Gain	Weight Neutral/Less Weight Gain	Weight Loss
Antidepressants	Lithium MAOIs Mirtazapine SNRIs SSRIs (paroxetine) TCAs (amitriptyline, doxepin, imipramine, nortriptyline)	SSRIs (fluoxetine, sertraline)	Bupropion
Antipsychotics	Clozapine Olanzapine Quetiapine Risperidone	Aripiprazole Lurasidone Ziprasidone	—
Antiepileptics	Carbamazepine Gabapentin Pregabalin Valproic acid	Lamotrigine Levetiracetam Phenytoin	Topiramate Zonisamide

Abbreviation: SNRI serotonin-norepinephrine reuptake inhibitors.
Adapted from Igel LI, Kumar RB, Saunders KH, et al. Practical Use of Pharmacotherapy for Obesity. Gastroenterology. 2017; 152(7):1765-1779; with permission.

adverse metabolic effects on lipids and/or insulin sensitivity, β-blockers can decrease metabolic rate by 10% and may have other negative effects on energy metabolism.[23]

In a meta-analysis of 8 prospective randomized controlled trials that lasted at least 6 months, changes in body weight were higher in individuals that received β-blocker treatment, with a median difference of 1.2 kg (range, −0.4–3.5 kg) between the β-blocker and the control group.[24] As a result, β-blockers should not necessarily be first-line treatment of hypertension in patients with overweight or obesity.

Not all β-blockers are associated with weight gain. Selective β-blockers with a vasodilating component such as carvedilol and nebivolol are recommended when β-blockers are required; for example, in patients with coronary artery disease, heart failure, or an arrhythmia.[3] These agents appear to have less potential for weight gain and minimally affect lipid and glucose metabolism.[25]

In a study of 1106 subjects with hypertension, patients taking metoprolol had a significant mean weight gain of 1.19 kg ($P<.001$) compared with patients taking carvedilol (mean weight gain of 0.17 kg; $P = .36$).[16,22] Although 4.5% of those assigned metoprolol gained at least 7% of their body weight, only 1.1% of those assigned carvedilol gained at least 7%.[22] This finding suggests that weight gain might be minimized by changing medications within the same class.

Antihypertensive medications that are not associated with weight gain or insulin resistance include angiotensin-converting enzyme (ACE) inhibitors, angiotensin receptor blockers (ARBs), and calcium channel blockers (CCBs). **Table 2** outlines specific antihypertensive medications associated with weight gain and weight neutrality.

Angiotensin contributes to obesity-related hypertension because it is overexpressed in obesity. As a result, ACE inhibitors and ARBs are desirable options for the treatment of patients with obesity. Because many patients with obesity also have prediabetes or type 2 diabetes, many of these patients could also benefit from the renal protection provided by these agents.

Table 2
Antihypertensive medications associated with weight gain and weight neutrality

Weight Gain	Weight Neutral
α-Adrenergic blockers	ACE inhibitors
β-Adrenergic blockers (atenolol, metoprolol, nadolol, propranolol)	ARBs
	β-Adrenergic blockers (carvedilol, nebivolol)
	CCBs
	Thiazides

From Saunders KH, Igel LI, Shukla AP, et al. Drug-induced weight gain: Rethinking our choices. J Fam Pract. 2016;65(11):780-788; with permission.

The Second Australian National Blood Pressure Trial, a prospective, randomized, open-label study of 6083 older subjects with hypertension, found that initiation of antihypertensive treatment involving ACE inhibitors in older subjects, particularly men, seems to lead to better cardiovascular outcomes than treatment with diuretic agents, despite similar reductions of blood pressure. Although thiazide diuretics are often recommended as first-line agents for the treatment of hypertension, their dose-related side effects, including dyslipidemia and insulin resistance, are undesirable in patients with obesity because they are prone to the metabolic syndrome and type 2 diabetes.

DIABETES MEDICATIONS

In a recent systematic review and meta-analysis of 257 randomized trials, weight gain was associated with the use of pioglitazone (2.6 kg), glimepiride (2.1 kg), glyburide (2.6 kg), glipizide (2.2 kg), and sitagliptin (0.55 kg). Weight loss was associated with the use of metformin (1.1 kg), acarbose (0.4 kg), miglitol (0.7 kg), pramlintide (2.3 kg), liraglutide (1.7 kg), and exenatide (1.2 kg).[5] **Table 3** reviews the weight profiles of several diabetes medications.

Sulfonylureas are associated with a mean weight gain of 1.5 to 2.5 kg.[26] In an analysis of 27 randomized controlled trials of noninsulin antidiabetic drugs in patients not controlled by metformin alone, thiazolidinediones, sulfonylureas, and meglitinides were associated with a 1.77 to 2.08 kg weight gain.[27] Furthermore, sulfonylureas and meglitinides were associated with higher rates of hypoglycemia than with placebo (relative risk range = 4.57–7.50). Sulfonylureas have the highest risk of serious hypoglycemia of any noninsulin therapy.[28]

Table 3
Antidiabetic medications associated with weight gain, weight neutrality, and weight loss

Weight Gain	Weight Neutral	Weight Loss
Insulin	α-Glucosidase inhibitors	GLP-1 agonists
Meglitinides	Bromocriptine	Metformin
Sulfonylureas	Colesevelam	Pramlintide
Thiazolidinediones	DPP-4 inhibitors	SGLT2 inhibitors

Abbreviations: DPP-4, dipeptidyl peptidase-4; GLP-1, glucagonlike peptide-1; SGLT2, sodium-glucose cotransporter 2.
   From Saunders KH, Igel LI, Shukla AP, et al. Drug-induced weight gain: Rethinking our choices. J Fam Pract. 2016;65(11):780-788; with permission.

Metformin, the most commonly prescribed oral agent for the treatment of type 2 diabetes, promotes mild weight loss by multiple mechanisms. These mechanisms include reduction of hepatic glucose production and intestinal absorption of glucose, as well as changes in hypothalamic physiology leading to leptin and insulin sensitivity.[29] There is also evidence that metformin decreases ghrelin levels and increases glucagonlike peptide-1 (GLP-1) levels, which further contribute to its anorectic effect. Given its efficacy as well as safety profile, some physicians are advocating its approval for the treatment of obesity.[20]

GLP-1 agonists mimic the gastrointestinal incretin hormone, GLP-1, which is released in response to food intake. They enhance glucose-dependent insulin secretion, suppress glucagon, and slow gastric emptying. In addition to improving glycemic control, GLP-1 agonists lead to weight loss by decreasing appetite and enhancing satiety. Liraglutide was approved by the FDA for chronic weight management in 2014 at a higher dosage (3.0 mg daily) than is available for diabetes (1.8 mg daily). Weight loss occurs with all of the agents in this class, with the weekly agent, semaglutide, seeming to be most effective.

Sodium-glucose cotransporter 2 (SGLT2) inhibitors are a newer class of medication that reduce glucose reabsorption by the kidneys leading to increased urinary glucose excretion. They may result in weight loss in addition to reduced hyperglycemia caused by the subsequent calorie loss through glycosuria.[30]

Both dipeptidyl peptidase IV (DPP-4) inhibitors and α-glucosidase inhibitors (AGIs) seem to be weight neutral or lead to minimal changes in weight.[31] Although the systematic review referenced earlier found a 0.55-kg weight gain associated with sitagliptin, most studies examining the weight effects of DPP-4 inhibitors report weight neutrality.[32] Pramlintide, the amylin analogue that is FDA approved for use in combination with existing insulin treatment, can prevent weight gain or lead to weight loss.[33]

For patients with type 2 diabetes and obesity who require insulin, the Endocrine Society Clinical Practice Guideline recommends concomitantly prescribing at least 1 weight loss–promoting medication (eg, metformin, GLP-1 agonists, SGLT2 inhibitors, or pramlintide) in order to mitigate associated weight gain caused by insulin.[25]

The 2016 Comprehensive Type 2 Diabetes Management Algorithm published by the American Association of Clinical Endocrinologists and American College of Endocrinology recommends initiation of diabetes therapies based on the risk of weight gain and the risk of inducing hypoglycemia among other attributes of the medications. Metformin is recommended as first-line therapy followed by a GLP-1 agonist or an SGLT2 inhibitor as second-line therapy.

ORAL CONTRACEPTIVES AND PROGESTATIONAL AGENTS

When oral contraceptive pills were originally formulated in the 1960s, they had higher doses of estrogen and progestin. High doses of estrogen can cause weight gain through an increase in appetite and fluid retention, so weight gain from oral contraceptive pills was common several years ago. Modern formulations of these pills contain much lower doses of hormones, making excess weight gain less likely, but some women still report this effect. Current studies report infrequent weight gain in the first 2 to 3 months that improves over time. Progesterone-based contraceptive methods such as subcutaneous implants have been associated with significant weight gain.[34] Progesterone-eluting intrauterine devices (IUDs) are associated with weight gain in less than 5% of women. In women with a propensity to retain water and have an increase in appetite on hormonal contraception, other medications, such as barrier methods and nonhormonal IUDs, can be considered.

SMOKING CESSATION

Smoking cessation can be considering a form of iatrogenic weight gain. Smokers have lower body weights than nonsmokers, and cessation of smoking is generally associated with weight gain. Two explanations have been offered for the effect of smoking on body weight: first, smoking is thermogenic; that is, the metabolic rate during the act of smoking is higher than when the person is not smoking. Second, smoking reduces hunger and changes taste perception so smokers tend to eat less.[35]

SUMMARY

There are multiple commonly prescribed medicines in several areas of medicine that may cause weight gain. The most common agents known to do this are antipsychotics, antidepressants, and antiepileptics. Insulin, insulin secretagogues, and antihypertensive medicines also lead to weight gain but can now be replaced or used at lower doses in conjunction with newer agents that are weight neutral or that can induce weight loss. In addition, glucocorticoids, progestational hormones and implants, and oral contraceptives may contribute to weight gain in certain patients. When treating iatrogenic obesity, specifically medication-induced weight gain, medications should not be changed or adjusted without consulting with the initial prescriber while also emphasizing the importance of a calorie-restricted diet and increased physical activity to treat the obesity.

DISCLOSURE

Dr R.B. Kumar is a speaker for Novo Nordisk and Jansen Pharmaceuticals. Dr R.B. Kumar is a consultant to Gelesis and reports holding shares of Vivus, Myos Corp, and Zafgen. Dr L.J. Aronne reports receiving consulting fees from and/or serving on advisory boards for Jamieson Laboratories, Pfizer, Novo Nordisk, Eisai, Real Appeal, Janssen, and Gelesis; receiving research funding from Aspire Bariatrics, Allurion, Eisai, AstraZeneca, Gelesis, Janssen, and Novo Nordisk; having equity interests in BMIQ, ERX, Zafgen, Gelesis, MYOS, and Jamieson Laboratories; and serving on a board of directors for BMIQ, MYOS, and Jamieson Laboratories.

REFERENCES

1. Apovian CM, Aronne L, Powell AG. Clinical management of obesity. West Islip (NY): Professional Communications, Inc.; 2015.
2. Saunders KH, Igel LI, Shukla AP, et al. Drug-induced weight gain: Rethinking our choices. J Fam Pract 2016;65(11):780–2, 784-786,788.
3. Vandenberghe F, Gholam-Rezaee M, Saigí-Morgui N, et al. Importance of early weight changes to predict long-term weight gain during psychotropic drug treatment. J Clin Psychiatry 2015;76(11):e1417–23.
4. Serretti A, Mandelli L. Antidepressants and body weight: a comprehensive review and meta-analysis. J Clin Psychiatry 2010;71(10):1259–72.
5. Domecq JP, Prutsky G, Leppin A, et al. Clinical review: drugs commonly associated with weight change: a systematic review and meta-analysis. J Clin Endocrinol Metab 2015;100(2):363–70.
6. Norris SL, Zhang X, Avenell A, et al. Pharmacotherapy for weight loss in adults with type 2 diabetes mellitus. Cochrane Database Syst Rev 2005;(1):CD004096.
7. Gadde KM, Xiong GL. Bupropion for weight reduction. Expert Rev Neurother 2007;7(1):17–24.

8. Gadde KM, Parker CB, Maner LG, et al. Bupropion for weight loss: an investigation of efficacy and tolerability in overweight and obese women. Obes Res 2001; 9:544–51.
9. Igel LI, Kumar RB, Saunders KH, et al. Practical use of pharmacotherapy for obesity. Gastroenterology 2017;152(7):1765–79.
10. Lieberman JA, Stroup TS, McEvoy JP, et al. Effectiveness of antipsychotic drugs in patients with chronic schizophrenia. N Engl J Med 2005;353:1209–23.
11. Fiedorowicz JG, Miller DD, Bishop JR, et al. Systematic review and meta-analysis of pharmacological interventions for weight gain from antipsychotics and mood stabilizers. Curr Psychiatry Rev 2012;8(1):25–36.
12. Allison DB, Casey DE. Antipsychotic-induced weight gain: a review of the literature. J Clin Psychiatry 2001;62(suppl 7):22–31.
13. Leucht S, Cipriani A, Spineli L, et al. Comparative efficacy and tolerability of 15 antipsychotic drugs in schizophrenia: a multiple-treatments meta-analysis. Lancet 2013;382(9896):951–62.
14. Himmerich H, Minkwitz J, Kirkby KC. Weight gain and metabolic changes during treatment with antipsychotics and antidepressants. Endocr Metab Immune Disord Drug Targets 2015;15(4):252–60.
15. Ratliff JC, Barber JA, Palmese LB, et al. Association of prescription H1 antihistamine use with obesity: results from the National Health and Nutrition Examination Survey. Obesity (Silver Spring) 2010;18:2398–400.
16. Baptista T. Body weight gain induced by antipsychotic drugs: mechanisms and management. Acta Psychiatr Scand 1999;100(1):3–16.
17. Verrotti A, D'Egidio C, Mohn A, et al. Weight gain following treatment with valproic acid: pathogenetic mechanisms and clinical implications. Obes Rev 2011;12: e32–43.
18. DeToledo JC, Toledo C, DeCerce J, et al. Changes in body weight with chronic, high-dose gabapentin therapy. Ther Drug Monit 1997;19:394–6.
19. Gaspari CN, Guerreiro CA. Modification in body weight associated with antiepileptic drugs. Arq Neuropsiquiatr 2010;68:277–81.
20. Igel LI, Sinha A, Saunders KH, et al. Metformin: an Old Therapy that Deserves a New Indication for the Treatment of Obesity. Curr Atheroscler Rep 2016;18(4):16.
21. Jesus C, Jesus I, Agius M. A review of the evidence for the use of metformin in the treatment of metabolic syndrome caused by antipsychotics. Psychiatr Danub 2015;27(Suppl 1):S489–91.
22. Messerli FH, Bell DS, Fonseca V, et al. Body weight changes with beta-blocker use: results from GEMINI. Am J Med 2007;120(7):610–5.
23. Pischon T, Sharma AM. Use of beta-blockers in obesity hypertension: potential role of weight gain. Obes Rev 2001;2(4):275–80.
24. Sharma AM, Pischon T, Hardt S, et al. Hypothesis: Beta-adrenergic receptor blockers and weight gain: A systematic analysis. Hypertension 2001;37(2):250–4.
25. Apovian CM, Aronne LJ, Bessesen DH, et al. Pharmacological management of obesity: an endocrine Society clinical practice guideline. J Clin Endocrinol Metab 2015;100(2):342–62.
26. Phung OJ, Scholle JM, Talwar M, et al. Effect of noninsulin antidiabetic drugs added to metformin therapy on glycemic control, weight gain, and hypoglycemia in type 2 diabetes. JAMA 2010;303:1410–8.
27. Kahn SE, Haffner SM, Heise MA, et al. Glycemic durability of rosiglitazone, metformin, or glyburide monotherapy. N Engl J Med 2006;355:2427–43.
28. Garber AJ, Abrahamson MJ, Barzilay JI, et al. Consensus statement by the American Association of Clinical Endocrinologists and American College of

Endocrinology on the comprehensive type 2 diabetes management algorithm – 2016 executive summary. Endocr Pract 2016;22(1):84–113.

29. Malin SK, Kashyap SR. Effects of metformin on weight loss: potential mechanisms. Curr Opin Endocrinol Diabetes Obes 2014;21(5):323–9.

30. Ferrannini E, Solini A. SGLT2 inhibition in diabetes mellitus: rationale and clinical prospects. Nat Rev Endocrinol 2012;8(8):495–502.

31. van de Laar FA, Lucassen PL, Akkermans RP, et al. Alpha-glucosidase inhibitors for patients with type 2 diabetes: results from a Cochrane systematic review and meta-analysis. Diabetes Care 2005;28(1):154–63.

32. Hong ES, Khang AR, Yoon JW, et al. Comparison between sitagliptin as add-on therapy to insulin and insulin dose-increase therapy in uncontrolled Korean type 2 diabetes: CSI study. Diabetes Obes Metab 2012;14(9):795–802.

33. Aronne L, Fujioka K, Aroda V, et al. Progressive reduction in body weight after treatment with the amylin analog pramlintide in obese subjects: a phase 2, randomized, placebo-controlled, dose-escalation study. J Clin Endocrinol Metab 2007;92(8):2977–83.

34. Bahamondes L, Del Castillo S, Tabares G, et al. Comparison of weight increase in users of depot medroxyprogesterone acetate and copper IUD up to 5 years. Contraception 2001;64(4):223–5.

35. Veldheer S, Yingst J, Zhu J, et al. Ten-year weight gain in smokers who quit, smokers who continued smoking and never smokers in the United States, NHANES 2003-2012. Int J Obes (Lond) 2015;39(12):1727–32.

Role of Commercial Weight-Loss Programs in Medical Management of Obesity

Kimberly A. Gudzune, MD, MPH[a,*], Jeanne M. Clark, MD, MPH[b]

KEYWORDS

- Weight reduction programs • Obesity • Treatment outcome

KEY POINTS

- The physician's role in obesity management can include referral to commercial weight-loss programs with published, peer-reviewed evidence demonstrating their efficacy and safety.
- Several commercial programs meet the guideline-recommended standards of intensity and contain evidence-based components, including lower-calorie diet, increased physical activity, and behavioral strategies.
- Among the guideline concordant programs, 4 programs have demonstrated 12-month weight-loss efficacy and safety: Weight Watchers, Jenny Craig, Medifast, and OPTIFAST.
- Physicians who elect to refer patients to commercial programs should apply an evidence-based strategy, such as the 5 As, when counseling patients. Frequent follow-up may be needed to support patients during their participation.

INTRODUCTION

Nearly 40% of US adults are obese,[1] and elevated body weight has been associated with increased risk of cardiovascular disease, type 2 diabetes mellitus, and certain cancers.[2] In addition to these health burdens, obesity costs the United States approximately $190 billion annually in health care expenditures and contributes to lost productivity in the workplace.[3,4] In 2013, the American Medical Association recognized obesity as a complex, chronic disease that requires medical attention.[5] Clinical trials of behavioral lifestyle interventions have demonstrated that weight loss can prevent or improve the control of several obesity-related chronic conditions.[6–8] In this article, the

[a] Department of Medicine, Johns Hopkins University School of Medicine, 2024 East Monument Street, Room 2-621, Baltimore, MD 21224, USA; [b] Department of Medicine, Johns Hopkins University School of Medicine, 2024 East Monument Street, Room 2-600, Baltimore, MD 21224, USA
* Corresponding author.
E-mail address: gudzune@jhu.edu
Twitter: @gudzune (K.A.G.); @jmclark_md (J.M.C.)

Endocrinol Metab Clin N Am 49 (2020) 275–287
https://doi.org/10.1016/j.ecl.2020.02.006
0889-8529/20/© 2020 Elsevier Inc. All rights reserved.

physician's role in weight management is discussed, along with the evidence for commercial weight-loss programs, and how these commercial programs may be integrated into clinical practice.

PHYSICIANS' ROLE IN THE MEDICAL MANAGEMENT OF OBESITY

Prior research has found that patients want their physician involved in their weight-loss plan,[9] and patients have greater weight-loss success when this occurs.[10] The rate of obesity counseling among physicians remains low,[11,12] which stems from multiple factors, including lack of time in the clinical setting, insufficient training about obesity, and low self-efficacy for weight management skills.[13–15] Physicians who face these barriers can still have an important role in obesity management, in particular, the referral to evidence-based obesity treatment services. In a randomized controlled trial (RCT) where physicians referred their patients to a behavioral weight-loss program, patients who rated their physicians as more helpful lost significantly more weight than those who did not rate their physicians highly in this regard.[9] After referral to such programs, evidence supports the physician's role, providing accountability and encouragement for patients during follow-up visits.[16]

ADULT WEIGHT MANAGEMENT GUIDELINES

Multiple organizations have produced guidelines outlining recommendations regarding the screening for and treatment of obesity among adults, including the American Heart Association/American College of Cardiology/The Obesity Society (AHA/ACC/TOS),[17] the American Association of Clinical Endocrinologists/American College of Endocrinology (AACE/ACE),[18] and US Preventive Services Task Force (USPSTF).[19] **Table 1** provides an overview of these recommendations. In general, these guidelines recommend that patients with obesity participate in an intensive, comprehensive lifestyle program that encourages lower-calorie diet and increased physical activity by using behavioral strategies. However, physicians may find it challenging to identify local programs meeting these requirements in their areas. In fact, a prior study found that only 19% of community-based weight-loss programs had high concordance with the AHA/ACC/TOS guidelines.[20] It may be also difficult for physicians to determine whether a program meets guideline criteria by relying on information available online. A study found that program intensity, dietary change, physical activity, and use of behavioral strategies were often not reported or were inadequately described on Web sites, although this information could be obtained during telephone interviews.[20] This information gap presents a challenge, because many physicians may not have the time to screen and call multiple weight-loss programs in their community to obtain this information.

PHYSICIAN REFERRAL TO COMMERCIAL WEIGHT-LOSS PROGRAMS

Commercial weight-loss programs are ubiquitous across the United States, and notably the recommendations from AHA/ACC/TOS state, "commercial-based programs that provide a comprehensive lifestyle intervention can be prescribed as an option for weight loss, provided there is peer-reviewed published evidence of their safety and efficacy."[17] In a trial, patients referred to a commercial weight-loss program by their physician lost twice as much weight as patients who only received weight-loss counseling from their primary care physician in the clinic setting.[21] An initial referral from the physician and subsequent follow-up visits helped emphasize to patients the medical relevance and health benefits of their participation in the program.[22]

Table 1
Overview of adult weight management recommendations from various US organizations

Organization	Year of Publication	Recommendation
American Heart Association, American College of Cardiology, and The Obesity Society (AHA/ACC/TOS)	2013	Patients with obesity enroll in a comprehensive lifestyle program for at least 6 mo that encourages a lower-calorie diet and increased physical activity by using behavioral strategies; the program should be high intensity, meaning that patients participate in at least 14 sessions in 6 mo.[17]
American Association of Clinical Endocrinologists and American College of Endocrinology (AACE/ACE)	2016	The treatment of obesity should be delivered by a multidisciplinary team and include a meal plan, increased physical activity, and behavior change strategies, such as self-monitoring, goal setting, and problem-solving.[18]
US Preventive Services Task Force (USPSTF)	2018	Adults with obesity should enroll in an intensive, multicomponent behavioral intervention for 12–24 mo that encourages lower-calorie diet, increased physical activity, and self-monitoring and provides tools to support weight loss.[19] The intensity should be at least 12 sessions in the first 12 mo.

Data from Refs.[17–19]

Some commercial programs include the recommended services and intensity suggested by guidelines (**Table 2**). Physicians considering referral to these programs should be familiar with which programs meet guideline criteria.

When relying on these programs to deliver behavioral interventions, the authors recommend that physicians still apply evidence-based counseling strategies that promote behavior change when discussing obesity and referral to commercial weight-loss programs. The 5 As: Assess, Advise, Agree, Assist, Arrange, can be a key strategy that physicians use for this purpose.[23–25] Prior studies have demonstrated that physician discussions that use the 5 As are associated with increased motivation to lose weight and greater patient weight-loss success.[26,27] **Table 3** provides an overview of the weight-loss counseling goals for each "A" as well as some example actions that physicians might take with patients during each step in regards to referral to a commercial program. Physicians who refer to these programs should be aware that 2-way communication between the commercial weight-loss program and the physician is typically limited. Therefore, proactively scheduling follow-up appointments, the first follow-up within 4 weeks and then at least every 3 months after that point, enables the physician to remain active in the process, provide continued support to the patient, and check in on lifestyle changes and weight loss. With weight-loss success, physicians will also need to use these follow-ups to monitor for the need for medication adjustments, such as decreasing the dose of antihypertensive medications as blood pressure decreases or modifying the medication regimen for patients with diabetes mellitus as their A1c and glucose improve.

Table 2
Outcomes and program components among guideline concordant commercial weight-loss programs[a]

Program	12-mo Weight-Loss Efficacy & Safety	Intensity[b]	Components			
			Nutrition	Physical Activity	Behavioral Strategies	Support
Weight Watchers	Yes	High	Low-calorie conventional food; points tracking	Activity tracking	Self-monitoring	Group session; online coaching; online forum
Jenny Craig	Yes	High	Low-calorie meal replacements	Encourages increased activity	Goal setting; self-monitoring	One-on-one counseling
Nutrisystem	No	High	Low-calorie meal replacements	Exercise plans	Self-monitoring	One-on-one counseling; online community forum
Medifast	Yes	High	Low-calorie meal replacements	Encourages increased activity	Self-monitoring	One-on-one counseling; online coaching
HMR	No	High	Low-calorie or lower-calorie meal replacements	Encourages increased activity	Goal setting	Group sessions; telephone coaching; medically supervised
OPTIFAST	Yes	High	Low-calorie or very-low-calorie meal replacements	Encourages increased activity	Problem-solving	One-on-one counseling; group support; medically supervised

[a] Information abstracted from program Web sites.
[b] High intensity defined as programs offering and recommending greater than 12 sessions per year.

Table 3		
Overview of the 5 As behavioral counseling approach and application to obesity		
5 A	**Goal for Weight-Loss Counseling**	**Possible Physician Actions Applicable to Commercial Weight-Loss Program Referral**
Assess	• Identifying appropriate patients for weight management	• Determine the patient's degree of obesity via body mass index • Determine cardiovascular and other risk factors • Assess readiness to change and readiness to participate in a commercial program
Advise	• Educating about health risks and benefits of change	• Educate the patient about his or her weight and the health risks linked with overweight and obesity • Weight loss can reduce blood pressure, improve cholesterol profile and blood sugar, and decrease risk of developing diabetes
Agree	• Collaborating to establish weight management goals	• Patient and physician agree upon goals ○ Goals should be quantifiable, achievable, and likely to lead to meaningful health benefits
Assist	• Determining the weight management strategy	• Review and referral to a guideline-concordant commercial weight-loss program with peer-reviewed published evidence of their safety and efficacy

Arrange	• Monitoring weight-loss progress	• Arrange first follow-up with the patient within 1 mo
		  ○ Provide accountability for patients, cheerlead their successes
		  ○ May need to adjust medications in response to weight-loss success
		• Continue to follow with the patient about weight loss after this visit at least once every 3 mo

The following sections of this article review this RCT evidence for the programs identified in **Table 2** that meet guideline recommendations with particular emphasis on weight and glycemic outcomes at 12 months.

WEIGHT WATCHERS

Weight Watchers is a high-intensity program in which individuals monitor their food intake by tracking "points" and their physical activity. This program is offered direct to consumers. Most of the RCTs of Weight Watchers have examined the in-person program, in which individuals attend group sessions on a weekly basis. Among these RCTs, Weight Watchers' participants achieved weight losses ranging from 3.6% to 7.3% of initial body weight at 6 months and 3.1% to 5.5% at 12 months.[28] These reductions were significantly greater than control groups at both time points.[29] A metaanalysis estimated that individuals participating in Weight Watchers lose 5.9 kg more than no diet at 12 months.[30] Of note, 1 RCT examined the efficacy of Weight Watchers Online (ie, no use of in-person groups) and found no significant difference in weight loss at 12 months compared with control.[31] Overall, no serious adverse events occurred or other harms were reported among Weight Watchers' participants within these trials.[29]

In addition to weight-loss outcomes, several of these RCTs have reported glycemic outcomes among Weight Watchers participants. Among individuals with euglycemia or prediabetes, Weight Watchers significantly lowered blood glucose or A1c more than the control group at 6 months; however, no significant between-group differences existed at 12 months.[32,33] Among patients with type 2 diabetes mellitus, 1 study found that Weight Watchers combined with diabetes education significantly lowered A1c at 12 months compared with standard diabetes support and education (A1c −0.3% vs +0.2%, respectively).[34]

A previous cost-effectiveness analysis identified Weight Watchers as the most cost-effective weight management strategy compared with other commercial programs.[35] Weight Watchers has low program fees as compared with other commercial programs; however, physicians should be aware that patients need to factor in their food costs to make a more appropriate price comparison with programs that use meal replacements, because the costs of these foods are included in the program fees. In summary, Weight Watchers has clear evidence to support its efficacy in safely achieving sustained, modest weight losses.

JENNY CRAIG

Jenny Craig is a high-intensity program in which individuals use meal replacements and are encouraged to increase their physical activity. This program is offered direct to consumers. Among RCTs that have examined Jenny Craig, participants achieved weight losses ranging from 7.8% to 10.0% of initial body weight at 6 months and from 7.1% to 10.9% at 12 months.[28] These reductions were significantly greater than control or counseling groups at both time points.[29] A metaanalysis estimated that individuals participating in Jenny Craig lose 6.4 kg more than no diet at 12 months.[30] With regards to safety outcomes, serious events were rare: 2 deaths occurred among Jenny Craig participants (unrelated to program participation) and 1 participant required cholecystectomy.[29]

Glycemic outcomes have not been reported for Jenny Craig among individuals with euglycemia or prediabetes. One RCT did test the effect of Jenny Craig among patients with type 2 diabetes, which showed that Jenny Craig produced significant A1c reductions (0.4% greater at 12 months) than a comparator counseling intervention.[32]

Jenny Craig has high monthly costs; however, these fees do include the meal replacements. Jenny Craig was examined in a previous cost-effectiveness analysis, which identified Weight Watchers as a more cost-effective weight management strategy compared with this program.[35] In summary, Jenny Craig has clear evidence to support its efficacy in safely achieving sustained, modest weight losses.

NUTRISYSTEM

Nutrisystem is a high-intensity program in which individuals use meal replacements and exercise plans. This program is offered direct to consumers. Among RCTs that have examined Nutrisystem, participants with type 2 diabetes mellitus achieved weight losses of 7.8% of initial body weight at 6 months,[28] which was significantly greater than a counseling comparator.[29] This same trial demonstrated that

Nutrisystem significantly reduced A1c 0.3% more than counseling at 6 months.[32] No trials have examined 6-month Nutrisystem outcomes in patients without diabetes mellitus, and no trials have examined 12-month outcomes of this program. With regards to safety outcomes, serious events were rare (urinary retention with hematuria and myocardial infarction unrelated to program participation).[29]

In summary, Nutrisystem has preliminary evidence regarding its short-term weight-loss efficacy, safety, and glycemic benefits, based on a single trial, which has reported outcomes with this program at 6 months. Additional RCTs of Nutrisystem that follow participants to 12 months or beyond are needed to consider routine referrals by clinicians.

MEDIFAST

Medifast is a high-intensity program in which individuals use meal replacements and are encouraged to increase their physical activity. This program is offered direct to consumers. Medifast participants achieved an average weight loss of 6.7% of initial weight at 6 months and 4.2% to 7.8% at 10 to 12 months.[28,36] In 1 RCT among individuals with euglycemia, Medifast significantly lowered fasting blood glucose 3.1 mg/dL more than education comparator at 6 months and 2.8 mg/dL at 12 months.[36] There have been no trials in individuals with type 2 diabetes. When reported, no serious adverse events had occurred among Medifast participants.[28,36]

Medifast has high monthly costs; however, these fees do include the meal replacements. In summary, Medifast has adequate evidence to support its efficacy in safely achieving sustained, modest weight losses.

HEALTH MANAGEMENT RESOURCES

Health management resources (HMR) is a high-intensity program in which individuals use meal replacements, different calorie options are available (low calorie: 1200–1500 calories daily, and lower calorie: <1200 calories daily), and are encouraged to increase their physical activity. HMR is frequently offered as part of a medically supervised weight-loss program. Among RCTs that have examined low-calorie HMR delivered in person, participants achieved weight losses ranging from 13.4% to 13.9% of initial body weight at 6 months.[28,37] HMR significantly lowered fasting blood glucose 10.4 mg/dL more than counseling at 6 months in 1 RCT among individuals with euglycemia.[32] No long-term trials have evaluated HMR, and no trials have reported outcomes in patients with diabetes. With regards to safety outcomes, no serious events were reported, although constipation occurred commonly (56% of participants).[29]

In summary, HMR has evidence supporting its short-term weight-loss efficacy, safety, and glycemic benefits, but long-term evidence is lacking. Clinicians should be aware that constipation occurs commonly among participants in this program. Additional RCTs examining long-term outcomes with HMR are needed to consider routine referrals by clinicians.

OPTIFAST

OPTIFAST is a high-intensity program in which individuals use meal replacements, different calorie options are available (low calorie: 1000–1500 calories daily, and very low calorie: ≤800 calories daily), and are encouraged to increase their physical activity. OPTIFAST is offered as part of a medically supervised weight-loss program. Among RCTs, OPTIFAST participants achieved weight losses ranging from 12.0% to

16.1% of initial weight at 6 months and 8.6% to 10.5% at 12 to 15 months.[28,38] OPTI-FAST participants with type 2 diabetes mellitus had lower A1c (0.3%) than a counseling comparator at 6 months.[32] Of note, most RCTs examined the very-low-calorie version of OPTIFAST. With regards to safety outcomes, serious adverse events were rare, although mild adverse events (eg, gastrointestinal symptoms, dizziness, headache) occur in approximately 10% of patients.[29,38]

OPTIFAST is a medically supervised weight-loss program that uses meal replacements, which can have high costs if not covered by insurance. In summary, OPTIFAST has adequate evidence to support its efficacy in safely achieving sustained, modest weight losses.

OTHER COMMERCIAL PROGRAMS

Other commercial weight-loss programs are available to patients, which may meet the criteria described in guidelines[17,19]: a high-intensity program that focuses on diet, physical activity, and behavioral strategies. The authors have identified the following programs that use these evidence-based strategies: Dukan Diet, Ideal Protein, iDiet, L.A. Weight Loss, Robard, Spark People, and TOPS (Taking Off Pounds Sensibly). However, no RCTs are known of among a general population of individuals with obesity that tests their weight-loss efficacy or safety,[29] although iDiet has been tested in worksites.[39]

In contrast, several other commercial programs do not meet guideline criteria because they are all self-directed; however, they do have RCTs demonstrating weight-loss efficacy: Atkins, Volumetrics, and The Zone. Atkins advises participants to eat a low-carbohydrate diet and increase physical activity. Volumetrics promotes eating less energy-dense foods to lose weight. The Zone encourages eating meals in which 40% of calories come from carbohydrates, 30% from protein, and 30% from fat. In a metaanalysis comparing these diets over a 12-month period to a no-diet comparator, Atkins resulted in a 6.4-kg greater weight loss, and both Volumetrics and The Zone resulted in a 6.0-kg greater weight loss.[30] Given their demonstrated weight-loss efficacy, self-directed programs, such as Atkins, Volumetrics, and The Zone, may be appropriate for some patients. In particular, physicians could consider recommending one of these programs to a motivated patient if the dietary strategy appeals to them. Books are available that outline these strategies that patients can be directed to read. If this approach is selected, physicians might consider more frequent follow-up with patients, such as monthly for 3 to 6 months, to help support behavior change.

The Ornish program is a cardiovascular disease risk reduction program that emphasizes a low-fat vegetarian diet, exercise, stress management, and group support, which has been tested in patients with preexisting coronary heart disease and has demonstrated weight-loss efficacy. In a metaanalysis comparing Ornish over a 12-month period to a no-diet comparator, Ornish resulted in a 6.6-kg greater weight loss.[30] Although this program would meet guideline criteria, physicians should be aware that Ornish does not consider itself to be a weight-loss program. Physicians may consider referring patients to an Ornish program, particularly if the patient has a history of coronary artery disease or other cardiovascular disease. Health insurance may cover participation in an Ornish program at a certified site. For example, Medicare covers participation in Ornish for patients with heart disease under intensive cardiac rehabilitation, and other commercial payers may also cover this program for beneficiaries who have or have risk factors for coronary heart disease.

Smartphone applications that support diet and physical activity changes are also increasingly popular (eg, My Fitness Pal, Lose It!, Noom). Clinicians should be aware that few have been tested in RCTs and when tested have shown minimal short-term weight-loss benefits.[29,40]

CHALLENGES FOR PATIENTS REGARDING COMMERCIAL WEIGHT-LOSS PROGRAMS

In addition to commercial programs' outcomes and safety, physicians should also be aware of challenges that patients may experience with participation in these programs. The authors highlight a few common issues in later discussion.

The most common challenge is cost. Commercial weight-loss programs can be expensive and may be unaffordable to some patients. Physicians should be aware that many commercial programs offer different options at different costs; however, the least expensive version of the program may not be the version that has demonstrated weight-loss efficacy in RCTs. For example, the version of Weight Watchers where individuals participate in weekly groups has demonstrated weight-loss efficacy, and this version is typically a more expensive option. Weight Watchers does offer a less expensive option where individuals just have access to their online tracking platform, but Weight Watchers Online only did not demonstrate weight-loss efficacy in the 1 RCT conducted.[31] Of note, offering multiple versions of the program is common across commercial programs, and not just limited to Weight Watchers. Patients should inquire with their health insurance company and their employer to determine whether a commercial weight-loss program may be a covered benefit to them or whether discounts or other incentives are offered to participate. For example, Medicaid in Tennessee (TennCare) covered Weight Watchers for their beneficiaries, and an evaluation of this program found that 20% of TennCare participants achieved a clinically significant weight loss of 5% or greater by participating in the program.[41]

Physicians should be aware of factors associated with early dropout from commercial weight-loss programs, which occurs commonly. For example, in an analysis of more than 60,000 Jenny Craig clients, 27% drop out at 4 weeks and 58% by 13 weeks.[42] A 2011 systematic review of in-person weight-loss intervention trials found the following factors associated with greater dropout: younger age, lower educational status, unrealistic weight-loss expectations, and less initial weight loss.[43] In a recent study among an employer-based commercial program, individuals who had one or more chronic conditions were more likely to drop out by 8 weeks.[44] For patients who have a chronic condition, physicians who refer to these programs should consider arranging follow-up within 2 weeks to help support their participation in the program and address any challenges that their chronic condition may impose on their participation. Given that failure to lose weight in the first month has also been associated with greater likelihood of early dropout,[44] physicians arranging follow-up with all referred patients within 4 weeks is prudent to help identify and support patients who may be struggling.

When considering referral, physicians should remember that commercial weight-loss programs may not appeal to all patients. First, male patients may have different perceptions about their weight and weight-loss strategies. Among a sample of US men, 48% perceived themselves as having the right weight despite being overweight.[45] Men are also less likely to participate in an organized weight-loss program, like a commercial program, as compared with women.[46] Second, patients with other dietary restrictions or dietary preferences may find participating in a commercial program more challenging. For example, needing to follow a low sodium diet to manage hypertension can be more difficult when using a program that relies on prepackaged foods as meal replacements, because the sodium content of those foods can vary widely.[47] Physicians should emphasize to these patients that they need to read the nutrition label on the program's foods and select those items that meet both their calorie and sodium goals.

Finally, availability of commercial weight-loss programs may vary by setting. Although the guideline concordant programs discussed in this article are generally available in all states, the number of locations may be limited, and distribution may differ between rural, suburban, and urban locations. Physicians should familiarize themselves with which commercial programs are available in their area to help guide patients' selection.

CHALLENGES REGARDING COMMERCIAL WEIGHT-LOSS PROGRAM EVIDENCE

There are several issues regarding the evidence base that physicians should understand when considering referring patients to these programs. First, few studies have directly compared commercial weight-loss programs, and there is limited evidence that any one of the commercial weight-loss programs has superior weight-loss results.[48] Given that a head-to-head trial of different programs is the only methodology appropriate for directly comparing programs, it cannot be determined whether 1 program produces greater weight loss than another. Second, physicians should be aware that many studies have a high risk of bias, particularly related to high study attrition,[29,32] and should consider this fact when interpreting the results and presenting this information to their patients. Finally, the outcomes achieved in these RCTs may overestimate the likely effect among patients, given that program fees were waived with study participation and study participants typically represent a motivated group. A recent evaluation of an academic medical weight management program suggests that individuals with access to insurance coverage for nonsurgical obesity treatment have lower levels of attrition and similar levels of participation and outcomes as those who pay out of pocket.[49] Therefore, the waiver of program fees may have decreased attrition in these trials, but is unlikely to have influenced individuals' participation in the program. Coverage of commercial weight-loss program fees by employers or insurers might be a strategy to reduce health care disparities for low-income individuals.

SUMMARY

In conclusion, national guidelines recommend identifying and treating patients with obesity, and several recognize that referral outside of the clinical setting to weight-loss programs, including to commercial weight-loss programs, is needed given the time and knowledge barriers physicians face. However, these programs should meet guideline-recommended standards of intensity (at least 12 visits per year) and encourage lower-calorie diet and increased physical activity by using behavioral strategies.[17–19] Several commercial weight-loss programs meet these criteria and have demonstrated consistent weight-loss efficacy and safety beyond 6 months in multiple RCTs, including Weight Watchers, Jenny Craig, Medifast, and OPTIFAST. More limited evidence exists with respect to glycemic benefits in these programs; however, Weight Watchers and Jenny Craig have preliminary evidence to support reduction in A1c among participants with diabetes mellitus at 12 months. Many other commercial programs exist that do not yet meet AHA/ACC/TOS, AACE/ACE, and USPSTF recommendations or have not yet demonstrated their efficacy and safety through published RCTs.

Thus, physicians might consider referral to Weight Watchers, Jenny Craig, Medifast, and OPTIFAST for their average patient who has obesity and is recommended to lose weight. For patients with obesity and diabetes mellitus, referral to Weight Watchers or Jenny Craig may be appropriate. Physicians should be aware that OPTIFAST, unlike the other programs, is offered as part of a medically supervised weight-loss program, and most evidence for OPTIFAST tests a very-low-calorie (800 calories per day) version of the program that may or may not be appropriate for all patients. Finally, physicians will also need to take into account patient preferences and finances during selection of a commercial weight-loss program.

DISCLOSURE

Dr K.A. Gudzune is a paid consultant for the American Board of Obesity Medicine and Eli Lilly. She is also supported by a grant from NIMH (P50MH115842). Dr J.M. Clark is supported by a grant from NIDDK (U01DK057149).

REFERENCES

1. Hales CM, Carroll MD, Fryar CD, et al. Prevalence of obesity among adults and youth: United States, 2015–2016. NCHS data brief, no 288. Hyattsville (MD): National Center for Health Statistics; 2017.
2. Flegal KM, Graubard BI, Williamson DF, et al. Cause-specific excess deaths associated with underweight, overweight, and obesity. JAMA 2007;298:2028–37.
3. Cawley J, Meyerhoefer C. The medical care costs of obesity: an instrumental variables approach. J Health Econ 2012;31:219–30.
4. Colditz GA. Economic costs of obesity. Am J Clin Nutr 1992;55:503S–7S.
5. Kyle TK, Dhurandhar EJ, Allison DB. Regarding obesity as a disease: evolving policies and their implications. Endocrinol Metab Clin North Am 2016;45:511–20.
6. Appel LJ, Champagne CM, Harsha DW, et al, Writing Group of the PREMIER Collaborative Research Group. Effects of comprehensive lifestyle modification on blood pressure control: main results of the PREMIER clinical trial. JAMA 2003;289:2083–93.
7. Knowler WC, Barrett-Connor E, Fowler SE, et al. Reduction in the incidence of type 2 diabetes with lifestyle intervention or metformin. N Engl J Med 2002;346:393–403.
8. Knowler WC, Fowler SE, Hamman RF, et al, Diabetes Prevention Program Research Group. 10-year follow-up of diabetes incidence and weight loss in the Diabetes Prevention Program Outcomes Study. Lancet 2009;374:1677–86.
9. Bennett WL, Wang NY, Gudzune KA, et al. Satisfaction with primary care provider involvement is associated with greater weight loss: results from the practice-based POWER trial. Patient Educ Couns 2015;98:1099–105.
10. Gudzune KA, Bennett WL, Cooper LA, et al. Perceived judgment about weight can negatively influence weight loss: a cross-sectional study of overweight and obese patients. Prev Med 2014;62:103–7.
11. McAlpine DD, Wilson AR. Trends in obesity-related counseling in primary care. Med Care 2007;45:322–9.
12. Bleich SN, Pickett-Blakley O, Cooper LA. Physician practice patterns of obesity diagnosis and weight-related counseling. Patient Educ Couns 2011;82:123–9.
13. Kushner RF. Barriers to providing nutrition counseling by physicians: a survey of primary care practitioners. Prev Med 1995;24:546–52.
14. Gudzune KA, Clark JM, Appel LJ, et al. Primary care providers' communication with patients during weight counseling: a focus group study. Patient Educ Couns 2012;89:152–7.

15. Bleich SN, Bennett WL, Gudzune KA, et al. National survey of US primary care physicians' perspectives about causes of obesity and solutions to improve care. BMJ Open 2012;2:e001871.

16. Bennett WL, Gudzune KA, Appel LJ, et al. Insights from the POWER practice-based weight loss trial: a focus group study on the PCP's role in weight management. J Gen Intern Med 2014;29:50–8.

17. Jensen MD, Ryan DH, Apovian CM, et al. 2013 AHA/ACC/TOS guideline for the management of overweight and obesity in adults: a report of the American College of Cardiology/American Heart Association Task Force on Practice Guidelines and The Obesity Society. Circulation 2014;129:S102–38.

18. Garvey WT, Mechanick JI, Brett EM, et al. American Association of Clinical Endocrinologists and American College of Endocrinology comprehensive clinical practice guidelines for medical care of patients with obesity. Endocr Pract 2016;22(Suppl 3):1–203.

19. US Preventive Services Task Force. Behavioral weight loss interventions to prevent obesity-related morbidity and mortality in adults: US Preventive Services Task Force recommendation statement. JAMA 2018;320:1163–71.

20. Bloom B, Mehta AK, Clark JM, et al. Guideline-concordant weight loss programs in an urban area are uncommon and difficult to identify through the internet. Obesity (Silver Spring) 2016;24:583–8.

21. Jebb SA, Ahern AL, Olson AD, et al. Primary care referral to a commercial provider for weight loss treatment versus standard care: a randomized controlled trial. Lancet 2011;378:1485–92.

22. Allen JT, Cohn SR, Ahern AL. Experiences of a commercial weight loss programme after primary care referral: a qualitative study. Br J Gen Pract 2015;65: e248–55.

23. Whitlock EP, Orleans CT, Pender N, et al. Evaluating primary care behavioral counseling interventions: an evidence-based approach. Am J Prev Med 2002; 22:267–84.

24. Serdula MK, Khan LK, Dietz WH. Weight loss counseling revisited. JAMA 2003; 289:1747–50.

25. Gudzune KA. Dietary and behavioral approaches in the management of obesity. Gastroenterol Clin North Am 2016;45:653–61.

26. Jay M, Gillespie C, Schlair S, et al. Physicians' use of the 5As in counseling obese patients: is the quality of counseling associated with patients' motivation and intention to lose weight? BMC Health Serv Res 2010;10:159.

27. Alexander SC, Cox ME, Boling Turner CL, et al. Do the five A's work when physicians counsel about weight loss? Fam Med 2011;43:179–84.

28. Gudzune KA, Clark JM. Commercial weight-loss programs. In: Wadden TA, Bray GE, editors. Handbook of obesity treatment. 2nd edition. New York: Guilford Press; 2018. p. 480–91.

29. Gudzune KA, Doshi RS, Mehta AK, et al. Efficacy of commercial weight loss programs: an updated systematic review. Ann Intern Med 2015;162:501–12.

30. Johnston BC, Kanters S, Bandayrel K, et al. Comparison of weight loss among named diet programs in overweight and obese adults: a meta-analysis. JAMA 2014;312:923–33.

31. Thomas JG, Raynor HA, Bond DS, et al. Weight loss in Weight Watchers Online with and without an activity tracking device compared to control: a randomized trial. Obesity (Silver Spring) 2017;25:1014–21.

32. Chaudhry ZW, Doshi RS, Mehta AK, et al. A systematic review of commercial weight loss programmes' effect on glycemic outcomes among overweight and

obese adults with and without type 2 diabetes mellitus. Obes Rev 2016;17: 758–69.

33. Marrero DG, Palmer KN, Phillips EO, et al. Comparison of commercial and self-initiated weight loss programs in people with prediabetes: a randomized control trial. Am J Public Health 2016;106:949–56.

34. O'Neil PM, Mill-Kovach K, Tuerk PW, et al. Randomized controlled trial of a nationally available weight control program tailored for adults with type 2 diabetes. Obesity (Silver Spring) 2016;24:2269–77.

35. Finkelstein EA, Kruger E. Meta- and cost-effectiveness analysis of commercial weight loss strategies. Obesity (Silver Spring) 2014;22:1942–51.

36. Shikany JM, Thomas AS, Beasley TM, et al. Randomized controlled trial of the Medifast 5 & 1 Plan for weight loss. Int J Obes 2013;37:1571–8.

37. Donnelly JE, Goetz J, Gibson C, et al. Equivalent weight loss for weight management programs delivered by phone and clinic. Obesity (Silver Spring) 2013;21: 1951–9.

38. Ard JD, Lewis KH, Rothberg A, et al. Effectiveness of a Total Meal Replacement Program (OPTIFAST Program) on weight loss: results from the OPTIWIN study. Obesity (Silver Spring) 2019;27:22–9.

39. Salinardi TC, Batra P, Roberts SB, et al. Lifestyle intervention reduces body weight and improves cardiometabolic risk factors in worksites. Am J Clin Nutr 2013;97:667–76.

40. Laing BY, Mangione CM, Tseng CH, et al. Effectiveness of a smartphone application for weight loss compared with usual care in overweight primary care patients: a randomized, controlled trial. Ann Intern Med 2014;161:S5–12.

41. Mitchell NS, Ellison MC, Hill JO, et al. Evaluation of the effectiveness of making Weight Watchers available to Tennessee Medicaid (TennCare) recipients. J Gen Intern Med 2013;28:12–7.

42. Finley CE, Barlow CE, Greenway FL, et al. Retention rates and weight loss in a commercial weight loss program. Int J Obes (Lond) 2006;31:292–8.

43. Moroshko I, Brennan L, O'Brien P. Predictors of dropout in weight loss interventions: a systematic review of the literature. Obes Rev 2011;12:912–34.

44. Alexander E, Tseng E, Durkin N, et al. Factors associated with early dropout in an employer-based commercial weight-loss program. Obes Sci Pract 2018;4: 545–53.

45. Yaemsiri S, Slining MM, Agarwal SK. Perceived weight status, overweight diagnosis, and weight control among US adults: the NHANES 2003-2008 Study. Int J Obes (Lond) 2011;35:1063–70.

46. Neumark-Sztainer D, Sherwood NE, French SA, et al. Weight control behaviors among adult men and women: cause for concern? Obes Res 1999;7:179–88.

47. Mehta AK, Doshi RS, Chaudhry ZW, et al. Benefits of commercial weight-loss programs on blood pressure and lipids: a systematic review. Prev Med 2016;90: 86–99.

48. Vakil RM, Doshi RS, Mehta AK, et al. Direct comparisons of commercial weight loss programs on weight, waist circumference, and blood pressure: a systematic review. BMC Public Health 2016;16:460.

49. Ard JD, Emery M, Cook M, et al. Skin in the game: does paying for obesity treatment out of pocket lead to better outcomes compared to insurance coverage? Obesity (Silver Spring) 2017;25:993–6.

Strategies for Physical Activity Interventions in the Treatment of Obesity

John M. Jakicic, PhD*, Renee J. Rogers, PhD,
Audrey M. Collins, MS, Ronald Jackson, MS

KEYWORDS

- Physical activity • Exercise • Sedentary behavior • Obesity • Weight control

KEY POINTS

- Physical activity is an important lifestyle behavior that contributes to body weight regulation, which includes attenuation of weight gain, and to treatment of obesity.
- At least 150 minutes per week of moderate-to-vigorous intensity physical activity may attenuate weight gain, which may contribute to the prevention of obesity.
- On average, physical activity contributes to approximately 2 to 3 kg of weight loss over a period of up to 6 months, and it can facilitate reductions in total body and visceral adiposity.
- Moderate-to-vigorous physical activity ranging from 200 to 300 minutes per week enhances long-term weight loss success and attenuates weight regain.

INTRODUCTION

There are worldwide public health concerns regarding the high prevalence rates for overweight and obesity in many countries throughout the world.[1] The prevalence of overweight (body mass index [BMI] ≥ 25 kg/m^2) is approximately 70% within the United States, with the prevalence of obesity (BMI of ≥ 30 kg/m^2) and severe obesity (BMI of ≥ 35 kg/m^2) being approximately 36% and 16%, respectively.[2] The concerns arise owing to the association between excess body weight and numerous chronic conditions, which may include cardiovascular disease, diabetes, some forms of cancer, musculoskeletal disorders, and others.[3,4]

Given the association between excess body weight and negative health consequences, there is a need for appropriate and effective options for the prevention and treatment of obesity. An important lifestyle factor that has been implicated for body weight regulation, attenuation of weight gain, and weight loss is physical activity.

Healthy Lifestyle Institute, University of Pittsburgh, 32 Oak Hill Court, Pittsburgh, PA 15261, USA
* Corresponding author.
E-mail address: jjakicic@pitt.edu
Twitter: @jmjakicic (J.M.J.); @ReneeJRogers (R.J.R.); @audcollins (A.M.C.)

Endocrinol Metab Clin N Am 49 (2020) 289–301
https://doi.org/10.1016/j.ecl.2020.02.004
0889-8529/20/© 2020 Elsevier Inc. All rights reserved.

This article provides an overview of key considerations related to the role of physical activity and strategies for engagement of patients in physical activity, within the context of body weight regulation and treatment for obesity.

PHYSICAL ACTIVITY FOR THE PREVENTION OF WEIGHT GAIN AND OBESITY

Given the high prevalence of overweight and obesity, it is important to focus efforts on weight loss and weight loss maintenance. However, from a public health perspective, it is also important to emphasize the need for efforts to prevent weight gain. The 2018 Physical Activity Guidelines Advisory Committee examined the evidence regarding the influence of physical activity on prevention of weight gain and the development of obesity.[5] Within the evidence reviewed, most studies showed an association between greater physical activity and attenuated weight gain. The evidence from prospective studies supports the potential importance of physical activity on the prevention of weight gain.[6–9] However, a relatively high level of physical activity may be necessary to demonstrate these effects. For example, Sims and colleagues[9] reported that moderate intensity physical activity equivalent to more than 167 minutes per week was protective against weight gain. When using a threshold of gaining at least 2 kg, Moholdt and colleagues[8] reported that achieving a threshold of either 150 minutes per week in moderate intensity or 60 minutes per week in vigorous intensity leisure time physical activity was protective against this magnitude of weight gain in men (relative risk [RR], 0.79; 95% confidence interval [CI], 0.69–0.91). However, the risk of gaining 2 kg was only decrease in women when physical activity exceeded the threshold of either 150 minutes per week in moderate intensity or 60 minutes per week in vigorous intensity leisure time physical activity (RR, 0.69; 95% CI, 0.59–0.82). In a study examining the odds of gaining at least 2 kg, Gebel and colleagues[7] reported a 10% decrease when a threshold of at least 300 minutes per week of moderate-to-vigorous intensity physical activity was achieved. It has also been shown that high levels of physical activity may be needed to decrease the odds of gaining 4.5 kg or more in women,[6] with 6 hours per week of moderate intensity physical activity decreasing the odds of this magnitude of weight gain (RR, 0.88; 95% CI, 0.77–0.99) compared with women engaging in less than 1.3 hours per week of moderate intensity physical activity.

In addition to evidence supporting that physical activity can prevent weight gain, there is evidence that physical activity can increase the odds of maintaining a healthy weight (ie, a BMI of $\geq$18.5 to <25 kg/m^2), with at least 166 minutes per week of moderate intensity physical activity demonstrating an effect.[10] There is also evidence that at least 1 to 2 hours per week of vigorous intensity physical activity can prevent the development of obesity in adult women.[11]

Thus, collectively, it seems that a relatively high amount of activity may be needed to minimize weight gain, or to maintain a healthy body weight, in adults. Based on the existing evidence, it also seems that the intensity of physical activity needs to be moderate or vigorous for there to be an effect on attenuation of weight gain, with limited data available for the influence of light intensity activity on attenuation of weight gain and the development of obesity.

PHYSICAL ACTIVITY WITHOUT DIETARY MODIFICATION FOR THE TREATMENT OF OBESITY

As described elsewhere in this article, physical activity has been associated with an attenuation of weight gain. However, there is also evidence that physical activity can contribute to weight loss.[4] A variety of modes of physical activity have been examined for their effects on weight loss that include cardiovascular (aerobic) activity, resistance activity, yoga, and lifestyle forms of physical activity, among others. However, when these forms of physical activity are undertaken without a concurrent decrease in energy intake, the effects on weight loss have been shown to typically be modest.

A review conducted for the 2008 Physical Activity Guidelines Advisory Committee Report showed that 180 to 270 minutes of physical activity per week can result in a weight loss of 0.5 to 3.0 kg.[12] This finding is consistent with the magnitude of weight loss reported by others in response to a 3- to 6-month intervention that did not include a prescribed reduction in energy intake,[13,14] and with clinical trials of longer duration.[15] However, a systematic review of the literature suggested that there may be a dose-response relationship between the amount of physical activity performed and the magnitude of weight loss observed.[16] For example, this review found that weight loss was 2.0 to 3.0 kg and 5.0 to 7.5 kg in response to greater than 150 and 225 to 420 minutes per week of physical activity, respectively. However, when activity was less than 150 minutes per week, there was no significant decrease in body weight. Thus, the dose of physical activity is an important consideration when developing interventions for weight loss that do not also include a prescribed reduction in energy intake, and the minimum threshold for physical activity may need to be at least 150 minutes per week.

Research has also been conducted to examine the effects of resistance training on weight loss. The interest in the role of resistance training for weight loss may stem from the potential for this form of physical activity to preserve or increase lean mass, and this may result in an increased resting metabolic rate, along with resistance exercise contributing to an increase in total daily energy expenditure.[16] Systematic reviews have demonstrated that resistance training seems to result in modest weight loss when not coupled with a prescribed reduction in energy intake,[16,17] with the majority of these data coming from short-term (<6 month) studies with limited data available from longer term studies.[16,17] The lack of a greater decrease in body weight may be due to a potential concomitant increase in lean mass that may result from resistance training.[18–21] Despite the modest weight loss observed with resistance training, this form of physical activity may result in a decrease in subcutaneous adipose tissue.[22] Moreover, resistance training results in improved strength and function. Collectively, data support that resistance training is a form of physical activity that can be beneficial for adults with obesity.

An alternative to structured forms of physical activity (eg, aerobic exercise, resistance training) is also lifestyle forms of physical activity that can result in an increased energy expenditure, and this has been termed nonexercise activity thermogenesis.[23] One approach to increase nonexercise activity thermogenesis is to encourage patients to engage in more walking episodes throughout the day, and this type of activity can be assessed with a pedometer or other activity monitoring device that detects steps walked. It has been shown that there can be a modest reduction in BMI (0.38 BMI units; equivalent to 2–3 kg of weight loss) with a consistent and sustained increase in physical activity by 2100 steps per day.[16] Moreover, an increase in 3000 steps per day has been shown to decrease waist circumference across a 12-week intervention period.[24] Thus, lifestyle forms of physical activity that are classified as nonexercise activity thermogenesis can provide modest decreases in weight and waist circumference.

Currently, a popular form of physical activity is yoga. A yoga practice consists of *asanas* (poses). These *asanas* can result in energy expenditure consistent with light-intensity physical activity (1.5 to <3.0 metabolic equivalents) when the *asanas* are performed in a restorative manner that simulates gentle movement patterns that are held before moving to the next movement.[25] The intensity of yoga can also be moderate to vigorous (eg, $\geq$3.0 metabolic equivalents) when the *asanas* flow in a dynamic and continuous manner, similar to a Vinyasa style of yoga.[26] Thus, this form of physical activity may have implications for attenuating weight gain or it may contribute to weight loss. Yoga may also include components of mindfulness meditation, which may influence stress, self-regulation, awareness, and psychological functioning and flexibility, and these may be factors that can impact weight and other health parameters in adults with obesity. However, the influence of yoga on weight gain prevention or weight loss has not been examined in appropriately designed intervention studies. Thus, recommending yoga for these purposes should be pursued with caution given the lack of scientific evidence in this area of study.

PHYSICAL ACTIVITY COMBINED WITH REDUCTIONS IN ENERGY INTAKE

Clinical guidelines for the treatment of obesity recommended that physical activity be combined with a decrease in energy intake.[4] Short-term studies (eg, $\leq$6 months in duration) typically demonstrate that adding physical activity to an energy-restricted diet results in an additional 2.0 to 3.0 kg of weight loss compared with what is observed in response to an energy restricted diet alone.[13,14,27] Although this magnitude of additional weight loss seems to be modest, this corresponds with approximately 20% more weight loss compared with what is observed with a dietary intervention alone.[28]

Beyond initial weight loss, physical activity seems to be an important lifestyle behavior for long-term weight loss maintenance and attenuating weight regain. There is a growing body of evidence to support that more than 200 to 300 minutes per week of moderate-to-vigorous intensity physical activity is associated with enhanced long-term (eg, 18–24 months) weight loss.[29–35] Although most of these studies have examined self-reported physical activity data when demonstrating these associations, there is now also a growing body of literature from objectively measured physical activity data to further support these conclusions. For example, 200 to 300 minutes per week of objectively measured moderate-to-vigorous physical activity performed in bouts of at least 10 minutes in duration has been shown to be associated with long-term weight loss.[36] Moreover, there is evidence to support that accumulating 10,000 steps per day, with approximately 3500 steps per day performed at a moderate-to-vigorous intensity, is associated with the ability to lose and maintain at least a 10% weight loss across a period of 18 months.[37] Thus, the evidence supports that physical activity is an important lifestyle target to enhance weight loss in adults with overweight or obesity, with additional evidence to support that a relatively high amount of physical activity (eg, 200–300 minutes per week) may be required to elicit these results.

PATHWAYS BY WHICH PHYSICAL ACTIVITY MAY INFLUENCE BODY WEIGHT

There is significant interindividual variability in body weight regulation resulting from physical activity.[38] In response to highly controlled exercise for a period of 4 months, 1 study reported that weight loss ranged from 3 to 12 kg.[39] Thus, it is important to consider factors that may contribute to this variability in weight in response to physical activity. These factors may include biological factors, the influence of physical activity on energy intake, and the influence of physical activity on energy expenditure.

In a study of multiple pairs of identical twins who engaged in structured and supervised physical activity, with energy intake held constant, it was reported that there was similar weight loss within a single twin pair; however, there was high variability in weight loss between pairs of twins.[40] These findings suggest that there may be biological factors that influence the effect of physical activity on body weight regulation.

The variability in body weight resulting from physical activity may also be influenced by its effects on components of energy balance (eg, energy intake and energy expenditure). For example, studies have demonstrated that approximately 50% of adults increase their energy intake in response to an acute bout of physical activity that ranges from 35 to 50 minutes in duration.[41,42] There also may also be an increase in resting metabolic rate in response to physical activity,[43] which can result in an overall increase in total daily energy expenditure. Thus, the influence of physical activity on components of energy balance should be considered with regard to the potential variability in body weight regulation. This finding may have clinical implications for approaches to preventing weight gain or to treating obesity.

STRATEGIES FOR ENHANCING PHYSICAL ACTIVITY ENGAGEMENT
Accumulation of Short Bouts of Physical Activity

There is emerging evidence to support that long, continuous periods of physical activity may not be required for health benefits, but rather physical activity could be accumulated across the day in shorter periods of time. This concept was endorsed by United States Centers for Disease Control and Prevention and the American College of Sports Medicine, and it was suggested that these periods of physical activity could be 8 to 10 minutes in duration, and that these short bouts of activity could be repeated numerous times throughout the day.[44] This paradigm was reinforced by other leading health organizations,[45] along with the *2008 Physical Activity Guidelines for Americans* stating that "aerobic activity should be performed in episodes of ≥10 minutes."[46]

Specific to body weight and obesity, results from prospective cohort studies support that physical activity should be accumulated in bouts of at least 10 minutes, and this pattern of physical activity is associated with a lower incidence of obesity.[47] This finding is further supported by intervention studies where moderate-to-vigorous physical activity performed in bouts of at least 10 minutes was associated with weight loss at both 6 months[48] and 18 months,[36] whereas physical activity accumulated in bouts of less than 10 minutes in duration was not associated with weight loss within the context of a comprehensive behavioral weight loss program. This finding may have implications for interventions to decrease body weight, and this strategy has also been shown to enhance physical activity participation in adults with obesity.[31,49]

More recently, the 2018 Physical Activity Guidelines Advisory Committee Report[5] examined whether physical activity accumulated in bouts less than 10 minutes in duration would elicit health benefits. Although the majority of the evidence available was from cross-sectional studies, there were data to support that physical activity accumulated throughout the day, regardless of bout length, was associated with a variety of health benefits. Thus, short bouts of activity such as climbing the stairs, parking further away from a store entrance, or other lifestyle forms of activity could be beneficial for health. However, with regard to weight and obesity-related measures, the evidence is mixed on the benefits of physical activity accumulated in bouts of less than 10 minutes in duration. Regardless, this contemporary paradigm shift may facilitate engagement in physical activity in adults with obesity, which may culminate in health-related benefits beyond weight loss that otherwise would not be realized.

Technology and Physical Activity

There has been an increase in commercially available technologies that have been applied to physical activity, with an increased emphasis on wearable technologies that monitor and provide feedback to participants regarding their physical activity behaviors. Thus, research has focused on examining the effects of these wearable technologies when applied within the context of weight control programs and other interventions targeting adults with obesity.

Studies have demonstrated a modest improvement in weight loss when a wearable physical activity technology was added to a weight loss intervention, with these studies typically being 3 to 9 months in duration.[50,51] Studies have also showed that when these devices are combined with a less intensive intervention (eg, less or no in-person contact with a weight loss counselor), effects on weight and physical activity were comparable with what was achieved with a more intensive program that involved regular in-person contact with a weight loss counselor.[52,53] These findings suggest that there are favorable effects of wearable technologies on physical activity and weight loss when applied within the context of a weight loss intervention for adults with obesity.

An additional approach that has been examined is combining wearable devices with other technologies. Patel and colleagues[54] combined a wearable device with a behavioral strategy focused on gamification, which incorporates game design elements, and examined the effects on physical activity in adults with overweight or obesity. The intervention was further enhanced by randomizing participants to 1 of 3 social incentive groups (support, collaboration, or competition), which were designed to further increase their physical activity across a 24-week intervention and a 12-week follow-up period. All 3 of these social incentive groups demonstrated a higher level of physical activity after the initial 24-week intervention compared with a control condition by 600 to 1000 additional steps per day. However, after the 12-week follow-up period, only the gamification intervention that included a wearable device combined with a competition element, which required participants to compete against each other toward higher levels of physical activity, resulted in a higher level of physical activity compared with control by approximately 600 additional steps per day.

Although these short-term studies show that wearable technology may be an effective strategy when applied to behavioral weight loss interventions, these findings should be interpreted with caution. Given the short-term duration of these studies, it is unclear whether the benefit on weight control will be sustained for a longer period of time, or whether there will be drop-off in the use of these technologies as intervention periods are extended. For example, Finkelstein and colleagues[55] reported that combining wearable technology with incentives for physical activity goal achievement enhanced the time that the activity monitor was worn and also the amount of physical activity over an initial 12-week period. However, when the incentives were removed at 12 weeks, both the use of the activity monitor and the amount of physical activity showed a dramatic decrease, which we term behavioral drop-off. Thus, the long-term use of these devices and the effects on weight control behaviors and weight loss are needed.

There are few long-term studies that have examined the effect of wearable technologies on weight loss in adults with overweight or obesity. One study that has been conducted applied wearable devices after an initial 6-month weight loss period to examine the effects on weight loss maintenance and prevention of weight regain.[56] In this study, Jakicic and colleagues[56] found that the addition of a wearable technology actually resulted in less overall weight loss across a 24-month period compared with participants who did not receive wearable technology. Thus, these findings may indicate that clinicians should be cautious when recommending that patients with overweight or obesity rely on wearable technology long-term in an effort to enhance weight loss and prevent weight regain.

Although there has been a proliferation of wearable devices to monitor and provide feedback on physical activity, the effectiveness of these devices to enhance physical activity participation in adults with overweight or obesity is not compelling. The majority of the evidence in this area is short term (eg, ≤6 months in duration), and the long-term studies that are available do not support a benefit of these technologies. Moreover, the 2018 Physical Activity Guidelines Advisory Committee Report concluded that these devices may be most effective for enhancing physical activity when combined with other behavioral strategies; however, even within this context the effects seem to be less compelling in adults with overweight or obesity.[5]

Supervised Versus Nonsupervised Interventions

Within the context of obesity, a strategy to consider is whether periods of physical activity need to be conducted in an exercise facility under the supervision of an exercise professional or whether self-directed nonsupervised physical activity can also be effective. Provided that there is not a medical reason that would require direct supervision by a qualified health or exercise professional, the evidence supports that self-directed nonsupervised physical activity can be as effective as supervised exercise within the context of an obesity treatment program. Andersen and colleagues[57] reported that 16 weeks of supervised physical activity performed within the context of a behavioral weight loss intervention did not result in greater weight loss compared with what was achieved with an identical behavioral program coupled with self-directed nonsupervised physical activity.

More recent evidence further supports this conclusion. Creasy and colleagues[58] compared supervised and self-directed nonsupervised forms of structured physical activity within the context of a behavioral weight loss intervention. There was no difference in weight loss achieved when the supervised physical activity intervention was compared with the self-directed nonsupervised physical activity intervention. These findings have implications for incorporating physical activity into weight management interventions, with results suggesting that physical activity does not need to be conducted within the context of a supervised setting. This finding may have implications for facilitating the adoption and maintenance of physical activity in adults undergoing treatment of obesity.

Timing of Physical Activity

The majority of the scientific evidence has focused on the volume and intensity of physical activity that may be associated with body weight regulation, which includes both weight gain prevention and weight loss for the treatment of overweight and obesity. However, more recent evidence suggests that the daily timing of when physical activity occurs may be an important consideration that can also influence body weight. In response to a 10-month supervised physical activity program of young adults with overweight or obesity, it was found that those participants who completed the majority of their prescribed physical activity early in the day (between 7 AM and 12:00 PM) had greater weight loss compared with those participants who completed the majority of their prescribed physical activity later in the day (3:00 PM–7:00 PM).[59] The mechanisms for these findings are not clearly apparent and warrant further investigation. However, these results may suggest that, when possible, adults seeking weight loss should engage in physical activity early in the day because this timing may enhance weight loss success.

Sedentary Behavior

More recently, there has been an enhanced focus on the influence of sedentary behavior on a variety of health-related outcomes. This topic was a focal point of the 2018 Physical Activity Guidelines Advisory Committee Report, and it was concluded that sedentary behavior has a negative impact on many health-related outcomes such as mortality and chronic conditions such as cardiovascular disease.[5] The data on the influence of sedentary behavior on body weight and obesity are less compelling. Prospective data have demonstrated that the association between total sedentary behavior and a 5-year change in either BMI or waist circumference was not statistically significant.[60] However, when sedentary behavior was examined in bouts of at least 10 minutes in duration, there were associations with greater increases in BMI and waist circumference. This finding may suggest that there is a need to decrease extended periods of sedentary behavior rather than overall sedentary behavior to prevent weight gain and obesity within the context of interventions.

Studies of sedentary behavior that have used isotemporal substitution modeling provide additional insight regarding the potential influence of sedentary behavior, and potential intervention targets, on obesity-related measures. For example, Buman and colleagues[61] reported that sedentary behavior that is replaced by moderate-to-vigorous physical activity results in a lower waist circumference; however, no effect was observed when sedentary behavior is replaced by less intense forms of physical activity (eg, standing/stationing activity, light intensity activity). Within the context of a comprehensive weight loss program that included a focus on both diet and physical activity, Jakicic and colleagues[48] reported that change in sedentary behavior was not predictive of 6-month weight loss, but rather an increase in moderate-to-vigorous physical activity performed in bouts of at least 10 minutes combined with an increase in light intensity physical activity were predictive of weight loss. These findings may suggest that, rather than interventions focusing on decreasing sedentary behavior, these interventions may be made more effective by targeting increasing engagement in moderate-to-vigorous physical activity along with encouraging additional increases in light intensity physical activity.

APPLICATION FOR HEALTH CARE PROFESSIONALS

The scientific evidence supports the importance of physical activity within the context of body weight regulation, which includes prevention of weight gain, weight loss, and attenuation of weight regain. It is also clear that there may be a need to achieve a threshold of physical activity at which these weight-related benefits can be realized by patients. Thus, it is important that health care professionals engage in conversations with patients about physical activity and consider appropriate and effective strategies to facilitate adoption and maintenance of sufficient amount of physical activity. The following key points are examples that should be considered by health care professionals when engaging in these discussions with patients.

1. When engaging in discussions with patients regarding physical activity, this discussion should not initially focus on the optimal dose of physical activity that is required for weight control purposes. Rather, this discussion may need to first focus on strategies to begin to achieve some additional level of physical activity that can progress over time to achieve a higher and more optimal level.

2. It is important to understand the types of physical activity that may be most enjoyed by individual patients and to also consider the activity that may be most feasible in their current lifestyle. For some patients, this process may be obtaining a fitness center membership and going to this facility 3 to 5 times per week. However, for others this may be cost prohibitive and inconvenient given their work and family responsibilities; therefore, a walk around the neighborhood after dinner may be more enjoyable and feasible. It is important that a health care professional first focus on identifying the feasible and enjoyable types of physical activity for each individual patient before attempting to have the patient engage in what the clinician perceives as the optimal form of physical activity.
3. There are reasons that patients are already not sufficiently active, and this may be due to them not enjoying certain forms of physical activity or other barriers. A health care professional should query the patient regarding their current and potential future barriers to physical activity, and to then address potential options for overcoming these barriers.
4. Even the most active of individuals will have things arise that may threaten their best intentions to engage in regular physical activity. Thus, assisting the patient in understanding that this can occur even when they are well-intended to be active is an important consideration. Moreover, within this context, assisting the patient to understand the importance of identifying the next opportunity to reengage in physical activity is an important step in the prevention of prolonged lapses in physical activity.

SUMMARY

Physical activity is an important lifestyle behavior that contributes to body weight regulation, which includes attention of weight gain and to treat obesity. It seems that at least 150 minutes per week of moderate-to-vigorous intensity physical activity is needed to significantly attenuate weight gain, which may prevent of the development of obesity. Although modest weight loss is observed in response to physical activity, this weight loss is clinically meaningful. Moreover, moderate-to-vigorous physical activity ranging from 200 to 300 minutes per week seems to be important for enhancing long-term weight loss success and for attenuating weight regain. However, there is limited evidence that solely engaging in light intensity physical activity or decreasing sedentary behavior will have a significant impact on body weight regulation, but rather the effect is observed when these are coupled with an increase in moderate-to-vigorous physical activity that is of a sufficient dose. Thus, strategies that have been shown to be effective for engaging and sustaining physical activity should be applied to interventions for body weight regulation that focus on either attenuation of weight gain or weight loss. From a clinical perspective, physical activity should be coupled with other important lifestyle behaviors (eg, appropriate energy intake, sleep) to enhance body weight regulation in individuals at risk for weight gain or for those with obesity seeking weight loss treatment.

DISCLOSURE

Dr J.M. Jakicic serves on the Scientific Advisory Board for WW (formerly Weight Watchers International, Inc.).

REFERENCES

1. Flegal KM, Kruszon-Moran D, Carroll MD, et al. Trends in obesity among adults in the United States, 2005 to 2014. JAMA 2016;315(21):2284–91.

2. National Center for Health Statistics. Health, United States, 2016: with chartbook on long-term trends in healthy 2017. Hyattsville (MD).

3. Jensen MD, Ryan DH, Apovian CM, et al. 2013 AHA/ACC/TOS guideline for the management of overweight and obesity in adults: a report of the American College of Cardiology/American Heart Association Task Force on Practice Guidelines and The Obesity Society. J Am Coll Cardiol 2014;63:2985–3023.

4. National Institutes of Health National Heart Lung and Blood Institute. Clinical guidelines on the identification, evaluation, and treatment of overweight and obesity in adults - the evidence report. Obes Res 1998;6(suppl.2). p. 67S–82S.

5. 2018 Physical Activity Guidelines Advisory Committee. 2018 Physical Activity Guidelines Advisory Committee Scientific Report. Washington, DC: Department of Health and Human Services; 2018. p. F5-1-F5-36.

6. Blanck HM, McCullough ML, Patel AV, et al. Sedentary behavior, recreational physical activity, and 7-year weight gain among postmenopausal U.S. women. Obesity 2007;15(6):1578–88.

7. Gebel K, Ding D, Bauman AE. Volume and intensity of physical activity in a large population-based cohort of middle-aged and older Australians: prospective relationships with weight gain and physical function. Prev Med 2014;60:131–3.

8. Moholdt T, Wisloff U, Lydersen S, et al. Current physical activity guidelines for health are insufficient to mitigate long-term weight gain: more data in the fitness versus fatness debate (The HUNT study, Norway). Br J Sports Med 2014;48(20): 1489–96.

9. Sims ST, Larson JC, Lamonte MJ, et al. Physical activity and body mass: changes in younger versus older postmenopausal women. Med Sci Sports Exerc 2012; 44(1):89–97.

10. Brown WJ, Kabir E, Clark BK, et al. Maintaining a healthy BMI. Data from a 16-year study of young Australian women. Am J Prev Med 2016;51(6):e165–78.

11. Rosenberg L, Kipping-Ruane KL, Boggs DA, et al. Physical activity and the incidence of obesity in young African-American women. Am J Prev Med 2013;45(3): 262–8.

12. US Department of Health and Human Services. Physical activity guidelines advisory committee report 2008 2008. Available at: http://www.health.gov/paguidelines/committeereport.aspx. Accessed January 19, 2009.

13. Hagan RD, Upton SJ, Wong L, et al. The effects of aerobic conditioning and/or calorie restriction in overweight men and women. Med Sci Sports Exerc 1986; 18(1):87–94.

14. Wing RR, Venditti EM, Jakicic JM, et al. Lifestyle intervention in overweight individuals with a family history of diabetes. Diabetes Care 1998;21(3):350–9.

15. Jakicic JM, Otto AD, Semler L, et al. Effect of physical activity on 18-month weight change in overweight adults. Obesity 2011;19:100–9.

16. Donnelly JE, Blair SN, Jakicic JM, et al. ACSM position stand on appropriate intervention strategies for weight loss and prevention of weight regain for adults. Med Sci Sports Exerc 2009;42(2):459–71.

17. Donnelly JE, Jakicic JM, Pronk NP, et al. Is resistance exercise effective for weight management? Evidenced Based Preventive Medicine 2003;1(1):21–9.

18. Hunter GR, Bryan DR, Wetzstein CJ, et al. Resistance training and intra-abdominal adipose tissue in older men and women. Med Sci Sports Exerc 2002;34(6):1023–8.

19. Hunter GR, Wetzstein CJ, Fields DA, et al. Resistance training increases total energy expenditure and free-living physical activity in older adults. J Appl Physiol 2000;89:977–84.

20. Olson TP, Dengel DR, Leon AS, et al. Changes in inflammatory biomarkers following one-year of moderate resistance exercise in overweight women. Int J Obes 2007;31:996–1003.
21. Schmitz KH, Jensen MD, Kugler KC, et al. Strength training for obesity prevention in midlife women. Int J Obes Relat Metab Disord 2003;27:326–33.
22. Janssen I, Ross R. Effects of sex on the change in visceral, subcutaneous adipose tissue and skeletal muscle in response to weight loss. Int J Obes Relat Metab Disord 1999;23:1035–46.
23. Levine JA, Vander Weg MW, Hill JO, et al. Non-exercise activity thermogenesis: the crouching tiger hidden dragon of societal weight gain. Arterioscler Thromb Vasc Biol 2006;26:729–36.
24. Chan CB, Ryan DA, Tudor-Locke C. Health benefits of a pedometer-based physical activity intervention in sedentary workers. Prev Med 2004;39:1215–22.
25. Hagins M, Moore W, Rundle A. Does practicing hatha yoga satisfy recommendations for intensity of physical activity which improves and maintains health and cardiovascular fitness? BMC Complement Altern Med 2007;7(40). https://doi.org/10.1186/1472-6882-1187-1140.
26. Sherman SA, Rogers RJ, Davis KK, et al. Energy expenditure in vinyasa yoga versus walking. J Phys Act Health 2017. https://doi.org/10.1123/jpah.2016-0548.
27. Goodpaster BH, DeLany JP, Otto AD, et al. Effects of diet and physical activity interventions on weight loss and cardiometabolic risk factors in severely obese adults: a randomized trial. JAMA 2010;304(16):1795–802.
28. Curioni CC, Lourenco PM. Long-term weight loss after diet and exercise: systematic review. Int J Obes 2005;29:1168–74.
29. Catenacci VA, Grunwald GK, Ingebrigtsen JP, et al. Physical activity patterns using accelerometry in the National Weight Control Registry. Obesity 2011;19:1163–70.
30. Jakicic JM, Marcus BH, Lang W, et al. Effect of exercise on 24-month weight loss in overweight women. Arch Intern Med 2008;168(14):1550–9.
31. Jakicic JM, Winters C, Lang W, et al. Effects of intermittent exercise and use of home exercise equipment on adherence, weight loss, and fitness in overweight women: a randomized trial. JAMA 1999;282(16):1554–60.
32. Jeffery RW, Wing RR, Sherwood NE, et al. Physical activity and weight loss: does prescribing higher physical activity goals improve outcome? Am J Clin Nutr 2003;78(4):684–9.
33. Klem ML, Wing RR, McGuire MT, et al. A descriptive study of individuals successful at long-term maintenance of substantial weight loss. Am J Clin Nutr 1997;66:239–46.
34. Schoeller DA, Shay K, Kushner RF. How much physical activity is needed to minimize weight gain in previously obese women. Am J Clin Nutr 1997;66:551–6.
35. Unick JL, Jakicic JM, Marcus BH. Contribution of behavior intervention components to 24 month weight loss. Med Sci Sports Exerc 2010;42(4):745–53.
36. Jakicic JM, Tate DF, Lang W, et al. Objective physical activity and weight loss in adults: the Step-Up randomized clinical trial. Obesity 2014;22:2284–92.
37. Creasy SA, Lang W, Tate DF, et al. Pattern of daily steps is associated with weight loss: secondary analysis from the Step-Up randomized trial. Obesity 2018;26(6):977–84.
38. Donnelly JE, Smith BK. Is exercise effective for weight loss with ad-libitum diet? Energy balance, compensation, and gender differences. Exerc Sport Sci Rev 2005;33(4):169–74.

39. Bouchard C, Tremblay A, Nadeau A, et al. Long-term exercise training and constant energy intake. 1: effect on body composition and selected metabolic variables. Int J Obes 1990;14:57–73.

40. Bouchard C, Tremblay A, Despres JP, et al. The response to exercise with constant energy intake in identical twins. Obes Res 1994;2:400–10.

41. Finlayson G, Bryant E, Blundell JE, et al. Acute compensatory eating following exercise is associated with implicit hedonic wanting for food. Physiol Behav 2009; 97(1):62–7.

42. Unick JL, Otto AD, Helsel D, et al. The acute effect of exercise on energy intake in overweight/obese women. Appetite 2010;55(3):413–9.

43. Tremblay A, Fontaine E, Poehlman ET, et al. The effect of exercise-training on resting metabolic rate in lean and moderately obese individuals. Int J Obes 1986;10:511–7.

44. Pate RR, Pratt M, Blair SN, et al. Physical activity and public health: a recommendation from the Centers for Disease and Prevention and the American College of Sports Medicine. JAMA 1995;273(5):402–7.

45. Haskell WL, Lee I-M, Pate RR, et al. Physical activity and public health: updated recommendation for adults from the American College of Sports Medicine and the American Heart Association. Med Sci Sports Exerc 2007;39(8):1423–34.

46. US Department of Health and Human Services. 2008 Physical activity guidelines for Americans, vol. 2009. Washington, DC: Department of Health and Human Services; 2008.

47. White DK, Pettee Gabriel K, Kim Y, et al. Do short spurts of physical activity benefit health? The CARDIA Study. Med Sci Sports Exerc 2015;47(11):2353–8.

48. Jakicic JM, King WC, Marcus MD, et al. Short-term weight loss with diet and physical activity in young adults: the IDEA study. Obesity 2015;23(12):2385–97.

49. Jakicic JM, Wing RR, Butler BA, et al. Prescribing exercise in multiple short bouts versus one continuous bout: effects on adherence, cardiorespiratory fitness, and weight loss in overweight women. Int J Obes 1995;19:893–901.

50. Polzien KM, Jakicic JM, Tate DF, et al. The efficacy of a technology-based system in a short-term behavioral weight loss intervention. Obesity 2007;15(4):825–30.

51. Shugar SL, Barry VW, Sui X, et al. Electronic feedback in a diet- and physical activity-based lifestyle intervention for weight loss: a randomized controlled trial. Int J Behav Nutr Phys Act 2011;8:41–9.

52. Pellegrini CA, Verba SD, Otto AD, et al. The comparison of a technology-based system and an in-person behavioral weight loss intervention. Obesity 2012; 20(2):356–63.

53. Rogers RJ, Lang W, Gibbs BB, et al. Comparison of a technology-based system and in-person behavioral weight loss intervention in adults with severe obesity. Obes Sci Pract 2016;2(1):3–12.

54. Patel MS, Small DS, Harrison JD, et al. Effectiveness of behaviorally designed gamification interventions with social incentives for increasing physical activity among overweight and obese adults across the United States: the STEP UP randomized clinical trial. JAMA Intern Med 2019;179(12):1624–32.

55. Finkelstein EA, Haaland BA, Bilger M, et al. Effectiveness of activity trackers with and without incentives to increase physical activity (TRIPPA): a randomised controlled trial. Lancet Diabetes Endocrinol 2016;4(12):983–95.

56. Jakicic JM, Davis KK, Rogers RJ, et al. Effect of wearable technology combined with a lifestyle intervention on long-term weight loss in the IDEA Study: a randomized clinical trial. JAMA 2016;316(11):1161–71.

57. Andersen R, Wadden T, Bartlett S, et al. Effects of lifestyle activity vs structured aerobic exercise in obese women: a randomized trial. JAMA 1999;281:335–40.
58. Creasy SA, Rogers RJ, Gibbs BB, et al. Effects of supervised and unsupervised physical activity programmes for weight loss. Obes Sci Pract 2017;3:143–52.
59. Willis EA, Creasy SA, Honas JJ, et al. The effects of exercise session timing on weight loss and components of energy balance: Midwest Exercise Trial. Int J Obes 2019. https://doi.org/10.1038/s41366-019-0409-x.
60. Barone Gibbs B, Pettee GK, Carnethon MR, et al. Sedentary time, physical activity, and adiposity: cross-sectional and longitudinal associations in CARDIA. Am J Prev Med 2017;53(6):764–71.
61. Buman MP, Winkler EAH, Kurka JM, et al. Reallocating time to sleep, sedentary behaviors, or active behaviors: associations with cardiovascular disease risk biomarkers, NHANES 2005-2006. Am J Epidemiol 2014;179(3):323–34.

Barriers and Solutions for Prescribing Obesity Pharmacotherapy

Ken Fujioka, MD, Samantha R. Harris, MD*

KEYWORDS

- Obesity • Pharmacotherapy • Weight loss • Barriers • Reimbursement

KEY POINTS

- Weight loss medications are often underutilized by candidates who qualify for their use, despite evidence that they offer increased benefits in weight loss compared with lifestyle interventions alone.
- Frequently cited reasons for not prescribing medications include lack of comfort, lack of familiarity with or knowledge of the medications, fear of medication side effects, or a belief that they provide little benefit in helping individuals lose weight.
- To overcome both the stigma associated with weight loss medications and discomfort in prescribing, there is a need to further educate providers about the potential benefits of these medications.
- The insurance coverage of weight loss medications is improving along with the emergence of a cash discount price. Subsequently, weight loss medications are becoming more affordable to the average patient.

INTRODUCTION

The history of weight loss medications is littered with medications that have been withdrawn from the market for safety reasons. Although the use of these medications was likely well-intentioned, their side effects were devastating. In the 1930s, 2,4-dinitrophenol (DNP) became a popular weight loss medication that was accidently discovered after French ammunition workers were unintentionally absorbing and inhaling DNP and trinitrophenol while working. The workers experienced hyperthermia with weight loss, as the DNP uncoupled mitochondrial oxidative phosphorylation from ATP generation (via futile cycling). It was seemingly an ideal weight loss drug, given the increased thermogenesis and rapid weight loss. However, patients would experience profuse sweating, tachycardia, and hyperthermia. Unfortunately, many patients

Division of Diabetes and Endocrinology, Scripps Clinic Medical Group, 12395 El Camino Real, Suite 317, San Diego, CA 92130, USA
* Corresponding author.
E-mail address: Harris.Samantha@scrippshealth.org

Endocrinol Metab Clin N Am 49 (2020) 303–314
https://doi.org/10.1016/j.ecl.2020.02.007
0889-8529/20/© 2020 Elsevier Inc. All rights reserved.
endo.theclinics.com

developed cataracts, agranulocytosis, and liver failure, with more than 60 reported fatalities. The drug was eventually removed from the market in 1938. Sadly, it is still available for purchase online by unregulated vendors who generally target bodybuilders.[1,2]

The most famous weight loss medication to be removed from the market was fenfluramine, which was part of the weight loss combination known as "Fen-Phen." In the 1990s, Weintraub and colleagues[3] showed impressive weight loss with the combination of fenfluramine, a nonselective serotonin agonist, and phentermine, a sympathomimetic. After this study was published, cash-based "Fen-Phen clinics" appeared on many street corners and in strip malls throughout the United States. The number of visits for obesity treatment skyrocketed, and prescriptions for Fen-Phen went from 1 to 2 million prescriptions yearly, to 10 to 12 million in 1997.[4]

In 1997, an article released by the *New England Journal of Medicine* described pathologic thickening of the heart valves leading to aortic and mitral valve insufficiency in patients on fenfluramine.[5] It was later determined that there are serotonin 2B receptors located on heart valves as well as in the lungs. Fenfluramine is a nonselective serotonin agonist that appeared to be stimulating these serotonin 2B receptors. This resulted in both thickening of the heart valves (with subsequent valvulopathy) and/or pulmonary hypertension. In 1997, fenfluramine was removed from US and European markets.[6]

The most recent medication to be removed was sibutramine. Sibutramine is a norepinephrine and serotonin reuptake inhibitor that was approved by the Food and Drug Administration (FDA) in 1997. Its use was not found to result in valvulopathy or pulmonary hypertension, but led to a small increase in blood pressure and pulse. This prompted regulatory agencies to require a rigorous Cardiovascular Outcomes Trial (CVOT) that was eventually completed and published in 2010. The results showed a higher rate of major adverse cardiovascular events in the sibutramine group (11.4%) versus the placebo group (10.0%), and the medication was subsequently withdrawn from the United States and Europe.[7]

With this checkered past, it is not surprising that health care providers (HCPs) would be hesitant to prescribe weight loss medications. Currently, there are hundreds of millions of Americans eligible for weight loss medications, yet only 0.7% to 2.0% are prescribed a weight loss medication.[8] Past history is likely not the sole reason for the impressively low usage of weight loss medications; there are multiple other barriers including the cost of weight loss medications, safety side effect profiles, and lack of comfort with their use by both the HCP and patient (**Box 1**).

Box 1
Reasons cited by health care providers for not prescribing weight loss medications

Fear of adverse events

Limited experience using weight loss medications

High cost or lack of insurance coverage of medications

Perceived lack of effectiveness of weight loss medications

Presumed lack of patient motivation to lose weight

Insufficient training or education in obesity medicine

Inadequate time to devote to obesity medicine during visits

Data from Refs.[11–14]

THE LANDSCAPE IS CHANGING

Between 2012 and 2014, there were 4 new medications approved for chronic, long-term management of excess weight. The scientific discovery preceding these medications was based on a greatly improved understanding of how humans regulate their body weight. Thus, the overall knowledge of both obesity and potential drug targets has improved considerably. In addition, the FDA now requires rigorous safety and CVOTs of all new weight loss medications. Currently, 2 of the newer medications have already completed their CVOT trials.

Many of these barriers are now being addressed with more advanced, evidence-based science. This article examines the barriers to using weight loss medications and addresses how HCPs can both navigate and overcome them.

PROVIDER BARRIERS TO OBESITY PHARMACOTHERAPY

Despite the availability of medications approved by the FDA for long-term weight management, fewer than 2% of eligible patients will receive a prescription for a weight loss medication.[9,10] Although this low number is increasing, there remain many barriers that likely reduce the utilization of weight loss medications (see **Box 1**).

One commonly cited barrier is simply a general discomfort when using weight loss medications. This is, in part, likely due to very limited experience and lack of education with this class of medications, which has likely also led HCPs to question the efficacy of weight loss medications.

Limited Education on Obesity

Historically, obesity and its treatment have been neglected topics in medical school curriculums. Medical students and residents in training have reported that they receive inadequate education in the counseling and treatment of obesity.[15] Despite recommendations by the National Academy of Sciences for a minimum of 25 hours of nutrition education for medical students, many medical schools still offer very little or no training on nutrition.[15,16] Physicians-in-training often fail to recognize obesity as a disease, and have very limited clinical exposure to treating obesity.[17]

In addition, because of the recent release of many weight loss medications over the past 7 years, many providers are not familiar with their indications for use, as well as the FDA-approved long-term duration of use. This fundamental deficit in hands-on treatment of obesity may explain why health care providers are currently unfamiliar and uncomfortable with prescribing weight loss medications.

Consequently, providers often feel ill-prepared and lack confidence in providing weight loss treatment to patients. In a survey in which 80% of providers did not offer weight loss medications to patients, 68% stated they agreed or strongly agreed with the statement that they would be more likely to prescribe medication if given formal training on proper administration and monitoring.[12] Another evaluation of provider attitudes on obesity pharmacotherapy showed that HCPs felt they had insufficient knowledge about available medications (72%), had a lack of available resources for prescribing (56%), or lacked training and skill related to overall obesity management (47%).[11]

Further efforts to increase knowledge and awareness of obesity and its treatment options in medical education appear to be improving. In the past few years, attendance has doubled or tripled at review courses in obesity medicine. Currently, providers have to seek out specific training forums to receive in-depth education on obesity as a disease and its pharmacotherapy treatment options. There is some anecdotal evidence that medical schools may be increasing the hours of education on nutrition and obesity. Although the future implication of this is unclear, it is reassuring.

Perceived Lack of Effectiveness of Anti-Obesity Drugs

HCPs are often under the impression that prescription weight loss medications are not efficacious. In a study examining HCP attitudes toward these medications, 83% of providers surveyed cited a lack of effectiveness as an important barrier to prescribing medications. The number of providers who perceived the various drugs to be effective was low; only 0% to 33% of providers felt a particular medication would be "effective" depending on the medication class.[11] In a large survey of HCPs, lifestyle interventions were felt to be more efficacious than weight loss medications. Of those surveyed, 81% felt that general improvement in diet was likely to be "completely effective" in the treatment of obesity, whereas only 30% reported that prescription weight loss medications were likely to be effective.[14] In another survey of primary care providers, only 10.6% agreed that medications are effective in weight loss.[13] Efficacy of weight loss medications in randomized, phase 3 studies is well defined with the 4 most recently approved medications[18,19] (**Fig. 1**).

In addition to a newly approved super absorbent hydrogel device, the 4 most recently approved medications will result in an average of 5% to 10% weight loss. This amount of weight loss is sufficient in yielding significant health benefits.[20] It is important to note that this is only the average weight loss, and clinicians can dramatically improve weight loss by continuing the medication only in patients who seem to respond well to the drug. If an HCP were to give a particular weight loss medication to 100 patients, approximately half of those patients would do very well, losing an average of 10% of their body weight. The remaining half would lose only 2% or 3%.

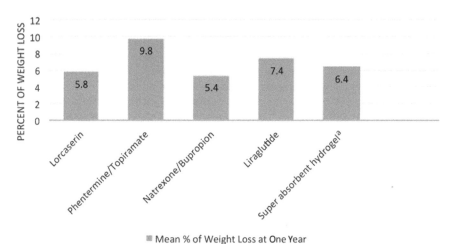

Mean % of Weight Loss at One Year

Fig. 1. Efficacy of weight loss medications. The older medications, phentermine and orlistat, are not included in this figure, as their weight loss has previously been well-documented, or, as in the case of phentermine, there is limited data on long-term use. [a] The recently approved super absorbent hydrogel is technically considered a device; however, it is consumed in pill form. (*Data from* Fujioka K. Current and emerging medications for overweight or obesity in people with comorbidities. Diabetes Obes Metab 2015;17(11):1021–32 and Greenway FL, Aronne LJ, Raben A, et al. A randomized, double-blind, placebo-controlled study of gelesis100: a novel nonsystemic oral hydrogel for weight loss. Obesity 2019;27(2):205–16.)

This is because weight loss medications have differing underlying mechanisms that correspond with the various causes of obesity. Thus, some patients are highly successful in losing weight on a particular medication and others are not.

Typically, the effectiveness of a particular medication can be assessed after 3 or 4 months of use. If the patient does not lose 4% to 5% of their total body weight within this period, the medication should be stopped, as the patient is considered a "nonresponder." This approach provides a simple trial for both providers and patients to evaluate if a particular medication is a good fit for the patient. The vast majority of patients who do lose 4% to 5% of their weight in this time frame typically go on to lose 10% or more of their weight. All of the newer medications have specific, more detailed guidelines to help clinicians identify medication responders and improve overall weight loss.[18,21,22]

Safety Profile of Weight Loss Medications

When HCPs are surveyed as to barriers to prescribing weight loss medications, "safety concerns" are often cited as the number one reason. The main underlying concern is the potential for adverse events related to the weight loss medication.[11,12] As mentioned earlier, this is not surprising, as there is a long history of weight loss medications being pulled from the market due to serious adverse events. This history has influenced the FDA to set a high bar for safety with regard to weight loss medications. Consequently, from 1998 to 2012, no new weight loss medications were approved. It was quite clear that pharmaceutical companies would have to demonstrate impressive safety data to obtain approval of any new weight loss medication.

Since 2012, 4 such medications have been approved. However, they were conditionally approved, and pharmaceutical companies are required to perform additional safety studies. The most robust and costly study is a CVOT. This type of study is specifically designed and powered to find any potential for the new medication to cause a cardiovascular event, such as a heart attack or stroke. These studies require large numbers of high-risk cardiovascular patients and years of follow-up to demonstrate that a particular weight loss medication is safe. A typical CVOT study will have more than 10,000 patients with diabetes and/or known underlying cardiovascular disease. The follow-up ranges from 3 to 5 years, and the typical cost is nearly a half billion dollars.

Of the 4 new weight loss medications, 2 have completed their CVOT studies (**Table 1**).

Lorcaserin recently completed its CVOT study in 2018 and was found to demonstrate cardiovascular safety.[23] Unfortunately, it was withdrawn from the market in early 2020 due to concerns for increased cancer risk. Liraglutide completed a CVOT in 2015 using the 1.8-mg dose that is approved for diabetes mellitus.[24] The 1.8-mg dose of liraglutide not only showed cardiovascular safety, but also demonstrated superior cardiovascular outcomes over placebo; hence the FDA allowed the previous CVOT trial to be used for the 3.0-mg dose used in obesity treatment. HCPs should feel very comfortable with the safety profile of liraglutide in high-risk cardiovascular patients.

The FDA uses another tool to ensure safety. It requires additional studies specific to the mechanism of the particular medication. An example is a weight loss drug that works via targeting the brain's serotonin receptor involved in satiety. In this scenario, the FDA would require additional studies looking at consequences of stimulating any serotonin receptor throughout the body. A pertinent example is the prior use of fenfluramine (the harmful component of Fen-Phen), which had a side effect of stimulating serotonin 2B receptors located on heart valves, leading

Table 1 Weight loss medications and CVOT results		
Medication	**Year CVOT Completed**	**Outcome**
Lorcaserin	2018	Safe: No significant difference vs placebo
Liraglutide 3.0 mg	2015	Safe: Superiority over placebo[a]
Phentermine/topiramate ER	Not completed	In discussions with FDA
Naltrexone/bupropion ER	Not completed	CVOT started but terminated early[b]

Abbreviations: CVOT, cardiovascular outcomes trial; FDA, Food and Drug Administration.
  [a] FDA allowed use of superiority data of liraglutide 1.8 mg, and liraglutide 3.0 mg was not required to do a CVOT.
  [b] After the company released interim CVOT data in a patent application, the executive committee of the study felt it became unblinded. The study was subsequently terminated.[25]
  Data from Bohula EA, Wiviott SD, McGuire DK, et al. Cardiovascular safety of lorcaserin in overweight or obese patients. N Engl J Med 2018;379(12):1107–17 and Marso SP, Daniels GH, Brown-Frandsen KB, LEADER Trial Investigators. Liraglutide and cardiovascular outcomes in type 2 diabetes. N Engl J Med 2016;374(4):311–22.

to valve hypertrophy and regurgitation.[5] This ultimately led to the removal of fenfluramine, a nonspecific serotonin receptor agonist. With this knowledge, lorcaserin, a specific serotonin 2C receptor agonist, was required to perform thousands of echocardiograms on patients taking the medication.[26] The FDA had to be assured that lorcaserin did not have any effects on the heart valves. Due to its specificity for the 2C receptor, lorcaserin was believed to have no effect on heart valves, and this was confirmed via echocardiographic imaging. The drug was subsequently approved for use by the FDA, though as previously mentioned, it has since been withdrawn from the market due to malignancy concerns.

Another route taken by pharmaceutical companies to develop safer weight loss drugs was to look at older, already approved medications that appear to have a side effect of weight loss. This was the approach used to develop 2 of the newer weight loss medications, natrexone/bupropion ER and phentermine/topiramate ER. The advantage of developing a weight loss medication using this strategy is that much of the safety data has already been produced. More importantly, millions of patients has already been on these approved medications and any safety issues ideally would already be well documented.

Finally, if a medication has the potential to benefit patients, but careful prescribing is needed, an educational system will be mandated by the FDA to improve its safe use. The system is known as a REMS program, or Risk Evaluation Mitigation Strategy, which is used to alert and educate HCPs, patients, and pharmacists of any potential problems. The newly approved medication phentermine/topiramate has a REMS identified, due to the potential for cleft lip or palate development in the fetus of mothers taking topiramate.[27,28] A REMS program educates patients and pharmacists, as well as HCPs, to ensure the female patient is informed to avoid pregnancy, and if she does conceive, to immediately stop the medication.[29]

In summary, the bar for approval of weight loss medications has become quite high due to the poor past history of weight loss medications. The safety studies now required of weight loss medications have been established to ensure that only safe medications are approved, and even more importantly, remain available for use. The 4 recent medications were approved in this "safety first" environment, and 2 of these medications have passed the most stringent of all safety trials (CVOT) with impressive results. With the safety issue addressed, the comfort level and use of anti-obesity medications are expected to increase.

Costs of Weight Loss Medications: Who Will Pay and What is Affordable?

Both patients and HCPs are concerned about insurance coverage and reimbursement for weight loss medications. Cost is usually cited as one of the top barriers for pre-scribing weight loss medications. More than 75% of HCPs saw cost as both a barrier (if the medication *was not* covered) and a "facilitator" if the medication *was* covered by insurance.[11,12]

For many patients, weight loss medications are not a covered benefit through insur-ance, and the patient will need to bear the out-of-pocket expense themselves. Unfor-tunately, the cost of some newer weight loss agents is often not within the budget of many patients. The lack of health insurance coverage of weight loss medications has been an ongoing problem for decades and is due to multiple issues that are discussed elsewhere in this article. Fortunately, this appears to be changing, and the insurance coverage of weight loss medications has been improving in recent years.

In a study looking at the proportion of state employee programs covering pharma-cotherapy for obesity treatment between 2009 and 2017, there was an impressive in-crease in coverage. In 2009, only 14 states covered pharmacotherapy; in 2017 this number jumped to 23 states.[30] This increase is a reflection of multiple changes within health care. As recently as 2010, fewer than 25% of insurance plans even tracked obesity, and "obesity" had not yet even been considered a disease in itself.[31,32]

In addition, the "payors" tended to hold on to the traditional belief that weight loss medications were ineffective and had adverse safety profiles. Fortunately, the issue of efficacy has been demonstrated in numerous phase 3 trials that meet the expectations of prescribing HCPs.[18,31] The safety concerns have also been addressed with recently completed CVOTs.[23,24]

The evolution of health care

The biggest change accounting for the improving coverage of weight loss medications has been within the health care system as a whole. Although it may be hard to believe, it is only recently that "obesity" has been defined as a chronic disease, which occurred via the passage of the Patient Protection and Affordable Care Act. This act will shift the financial incentives toward the treatment of obesity, as there are a high number of co-morbid diseases, with an associated cost burden, that can improve with weight loss.[33]

With the continuing advancements in safety and efficacy, and the evolving land-scape of medicine, the only remaining data needed is evidence of decreased health care costs with the use of weight loss medications. The Look AHEAD trial is a study considered by many to be one of the most significant studies examining weight loss in patients with obesity and diabetes. It used intensive lifestyle intervention to achieve at least 5% to 10% weight loss in participants. The study showed impressive and sta-tistically significant savings in health care costs. The 5% to 10% of weight loss achieved in this study is well within the range that can be expected from weight loss medications.[34] Hopefully, moving forward there will be more data to suggest cost improvements when weight loss medications are used.

Insurance coverage of weight loss medications

Currently, Medicare does not cover weight loss medications, but many state Medicaid programs and commercial insurance programs do provide coverage (**Table 2**).[35]

A recent study in 2018 looked at the state-by-state coverage of Medicare, Medicaid, and the Affordable Care Act (ACA) marketplace insurances. It was again shown that

Table 2

Table 2
Insurance coverage of weight loss medications

Medication	Commercial, %	Medicare, %	State Medicaid, %
Phentermine	53	0	60
Liraglutide 3.0 mg	57	0	62
Naltrexone 32 mg/Bupropion 360 mg ER	46	0	50
Lorcaserin	55	0	49
Phentermine 7.5 mg/Topiramate 46 mg ER	34	0	52

Data from MMIT formulary search for desktops. Available at: https://info.mmitnetwork.com/formulary. Accessed May 27, 2019.

weight loss medications lack coverage by Medicare. Of the 34 states that had available data, 8 states had some coverage of obesity medications. Looking at ACA health insurance, 9 of the 34 states had some type of coverage for obesity medications.[36]

The variability in coverage of medications is often a reflection of the employer that is purchasing the health coverage. Employers can opt out of covering weight loss medications to save on the cost of health insurance for their employees. This leads to differences in weight loss medication benefits, depending on both the location and employer that is purchasing the health insurance. In some areas of the United States, most patients have coverage for these medications, whereas in other regions, there is only a small percentage of patients with coverage.

HCPs should not hesitate to write a prescription for obesity medication because of fear of cost. There will be many instances when there is unexpected coverage of the medication. If a prior authorization (PA) is required, it is highly advisable to include the patient's body mass index and related medical conditions. Another important piece of information to be included relates to the patient's past history of weight loss attempts. If the patient has tried weight loss with diet and exercise for at least 6 months in the past, this should be included in the PA. This can include 6 months of visits with dietitians, commercial weight loss programs such as Weight Watchers, or even physician-supervised programs. Last, it is advisable to convey in the PA that the prescriber will regularly follow the patient and that the patient will continue appropriate dietary and lifestyle efforts.

As stated previously, based on the insurer and/or the employer, there may be some undesirable burdens associated with the administrative task of obtaining coverage for weight loss medications. Although this is unfortunate, these issues can often be reduced or eliminated by streamlining the PA process, that is, having designated office staff well-versed in local medication coverage and PA specifications. It is important to set realistic cost expectations with patients early on, which may include providing a cost-savings coupon card upfront, in case the patient will need to pay out-of-pocket. These strategies may be useful in overcoming coverage issues and can minimize delays in starting obesity pharmacotherapy.

Cash discount cards
There is another potential option for obtaining weight loss medications; in situations in which there is noncoverage of the medication, many pharmaceutical companies will give a discounted price to patients who pay out-of-pocket. The discounted prices of the newer medications are approximately $100 to $135 per month. Per data, this price is consistent with the amount patients are willing to pay. An online survey of the "willingness of patients to pay for obesity pharmacotherapy" has determined

that patients are willing to pay £6.51/$10.49 per month per percentage point of weight loss that a pharmacotherapy could provide.[37]

Overall, this equates to approximately $105 per month for an expected 10% weight loss. This suggests that the vast majority of patients who do not have coverage of weight loss medications are willing to pay the discounted price. **Table 3** shows the costs of the newer weight loss agents and their discounted prices.

In summary, insurance coverage of weight loss medications is improving at all levels. HCPs should not hesitate to write a prescription for a weight loss agent, as there is a reasonable probability that it will be covered.[33] If the weight loss medication is not covered, the patient can use the cash discount card provided by the pharmaceutical company and "pay cash" for the weight loss medication at an affordable cost of approximately $100 US dollars per month.

DISCUSSION ON OVERCOMING HEALTH CARE PROVIDER BARRIERS

The barriers of safety and efficacy are both falling rapidly, as 3 of the 4 recently approved medications have shown adequate efficacy as well as safety. The future is quite promising for the newer medications in development, which show even more impressive weight loss results. Glucagon-like peptide-1, gastric inhibitory peptide, and other hormonal treatments have presented the possibility of projected weight loss of 15% to 20%, which begins to rival the weight loss seen in bariatric surgery.[38–40] In terms of safety, the FDA has set a high bar for new drug approval, and HCPs can feel confident in the use of weight loss medications.

The cost of weight loss medications will always be an issue, but this appears to be improving. There is clearly more insurance coverage of weight loss medications, and HCPs should not hesitate to prescribe the medication to determine coverage. Benefits, including payment for these medications, can vary greatly between the different US states and regions. Although these authors admit it can be frustrating when multiple attempts to get a medication covered fail, it is noted that many do eventually succeed at obtaining coverage. Fortunately, even if the insurer does not cover the medication, many pharmaceutical companies offer a cash discount that most patients are willing to pay.

Education, experience, and comfort are the last barriers that are slowly coming down. Fortunately, both the interest and desire to learn about obesity medicine is

Table 3
Out-of-pocket medication cost with and without discount per month

Medication	Cash Price	Discounted Cash Price if Not Covered by Insurance
Orlistat 60mg (OTC)	$60	Not applicable
Phentermine 8mg[a]	$30-50	$20-30
Phentermine 37.5mg[a]	$15	$15
Phentermine 7.5mg/ Topiramate 46mg ER	$200	$100-130[b]
Naltrexone 32mg/ Bupropion 360mg ER	$282	$100-130[b]
Liraglutide 3.0mg	$1,500	$1,200

Approximate costs of a one-month supply of above weight loss medications based on internet pricing as of April 24, 2020.
Abbreviation: OTC, over the counter.
[a] Not approved for chronic long term use.
[b] Lower cost may require use of a specific mail-order pharmacy.

high, which has led to more conferences on obesity medicine. HCPs can choose from symposiums dedicated solely to obesity or attend larger annual conferences of numerous specialties, which have added sections devoted entirely to obesity management. Perhaps the most welcome change has been the dramatic increase in HCPs seeking certification by the American Board of Obesity Medicine. In 2019, more than 720 physicians passed the certification examination, which is 27% more providers than in 2018, bringing the total number of certified Obesity Medicine physicians to more than 3370.[41] This provides the HCP who is uncomfortable treating patients with obesity the option to refer the patient to a weight management specialist.

Given the complexities of obesity and the need for more intense interventions beyond lifestyle counseling, all potential solutions to its treatment should be considered to increase the likelihood of successful long-term weight loss.

DISCLOSURE

K. Fujioka has served as a paid consultant for Novo Nordisk, Eisai, Gelesis, KVK-tech, Amgen, Sunovion, Phenomix, Boehringer Ingelheim, Janssen Global Services, and Roivant; has received research funding from Eisai; and has been a speaker for Novo Nordisk. S.R. Harris has served as a paid consultant for Sanofi; has received research funding from Eisai; and has been a speaker for Valeritas.

REFERENCES

1. Holborow A, Purnell RM, Wong JF. Beware the yellow slimming pill: fatal 2,4-dinitrophenol overdose. BMJ Case Rep 2016. https://doi.org/10.1136/bcr-2016-214689.

2. Greenway FL, Caruso MK. Safety of obesity drugs. Expert Opin Drug Saf 2005; 4(6):1–13.

3. Weintraub M, Sundaresan PR, Madan M, et al. Long-term weight control study. I (weeks 0 to 34). The enhancement of behavior modification, caloric restriction, and exercise by fenfluramine plus phentermine versus placebo. Clin Pharmacol Ther 1992;51:586–94.

4. IMS Health, National Prescription Audit *Plus7*, Years 1997 – 2003, Extracted March 2004, NPA *Plus* Therapeutic Category Report, Years December 1966 -1996, Hard Copy Books.

5. Connolly H, Crary J, Mcgoon M, et al. Valvular heart disease associated with fenfluramine–phentermine. N Engl J Med 1997;337:581–8.

6. Krentz AJ, Fujioka K, Hompesch M. Evolution of pharmacological obesity treatments: focus on adverse side-effect profiles. Diabetes Obes Metab 2016;18: 558–70.

7. James WP, Caterson ID, Coutinho W, et al. Effect of sibutramine on cardiovascular outcomes in overweight and obese subjects. N Engl J Med 2010;363(10): 905–17.

8. Petrin C, Kahan S, Turner M, et al. Current practices of obesity pharmacotherapy, bariatric surgery referral and coding for counselling by healthcare professionals. Obes Sci Pract 2016;2(3):266–71.

9. Zhang S, Manne S, Lin J, et al. Characteristics of patients potentially eligible for pharmacotherapy for weight loss in primary care practice in the United States. Obes Sci Pract 2016;2:104–14.

10. Xia Y, Kelton CM, Guo JJ, et al. Treatment of obesity: pharmacotherapy trends in the United States from 1999 to 2010. Obesity 2015;23:1721–8.

11. Granara B, Laurent J. Provider attitudes and practice patterns of obesity management with pharmacotherapy. J Am Assoc Nurse Pract 2017;29(9):543–50.
12. Simon R, Lahiri SW. Provider practice habits and barriers to care in obesity management in a large multicenter health system. Endocr Pract 2018;24(4):321–8.
13. Salinas GD, Glauser TA, Williamson JC, et al. Primary care and physician attitudes and practice patterns in the management of obese adults: results from a national survey. Postgrad Med 2011;123(5):214–9.
14. Kaplan LM, Golden A, Jinnett K, et al. Perceptions of barriers to effective obesity care: results from the national ACTION study. Obesity 2018;26:61–9.
15. Danek RL, Berlin KL, Waite GN, et al. Perceptions of nutrition education in the current medical school curriculum. Fam Med 2017;49(10):803–6.
16. Adams KM, Kohlmeier M, Zeisel SH. Nutrition education in US medical schools: latest update of a national survey. Acad Med 2010;85:1537–42.
17. Metcalf M, Rossie K, Stokes K, et al. The perceptions of medical school students and faculty toward obesity medicine education: survey and needs analysis. JMIR Med Educ 2017;3(2):e22.
18. Fujioka K. Current and emerging medications for overweight or obesity in people with comorbidities. Diabetes Obes Metab 2015;17(11):1021–32.
19. Greenway FL, Aronne LJ, Raben A, et al. A randomized, double-blind, placebo-controlled study of gelesis100: a novel nonsystemic oral hydrogel for weight loss. Obesity 2019;27(2):205–16.
20. Yanovski SZ, Yanovski JA. Long-term drug treatment for obesity: a systematic and clinical review. JAMA 2014;311(1):74–86.
21. Fujioka K, O'Neil PM, Davies M, et al. Early weight loss with liraglutide 3.0 mg predicts 1-year weight loss and is associated with improvements in clinical markers. Obesity 2016;24(11):2278–88.
22. Fujioka K, Plodkowski R, O'Neil PM, et al. The relationship between early weight loss and weight loss at 1 year with naltrexone ER/bupropion ER combination therapy. Int J Obes 2016;40(9):1369–75.
23. Bohula EA, Wiviott SD, McGuire DK, et al. Cardiovascular safety of lorcaserin in overweight or obese patients. N Engl J Med 2018;379(12):1107–17.
24. Marso SP, Daniels GH, Brown-Frandsen KB, LEADER Trial Investigators. Liraglutide and cardiovascular outcomes in type 2 diabetes. N Engl J Med 2016;374(4): 311–22.
25. CardioBrief: diet drug loses another cardiovascular outcomes trial – More chaos over the weight loss drug Contrave. Medpage Today in collaboration with AACE. 2016. Available at: https://www.medpagetoday.com/cardiology/cardiobrief/ 57339. Accessed July 8, 2019.
26. Weissman NJ, Sanchez M, Koch GG, et al. Echocardiographic assessment of cardiac valvular regurgitation with lorcaserin from analysis of 3 phase 3 clinical trials. Circ Cardiovasc Imaging 2013;6:560–7.
27. Fujioka K. Safety and tolerability of medications approved for chronic weight management. Obesity 2015;23(1):S7–11.
28. Colman E, Golden J, Roberts M, et al. The FDA's assessment of two drugs for chronic weight management. N Engl J Med 2012;367(17):1577–9.
29. Qsymia™ (Phentermine/topiramate ER) product REMS. U.S. Food & Drug Administration Website. 2013. Available at: https://www.fda.gov/media/86139/ download. Accessed August 2, 2019.
30. Jannah N, Hild J, Gallagher C, et al. Coverage for obesity prevention and treatment services: analysis of Medicaid and state employee health insurance programs. Obesity 2018;26(12):1834–40.

31. Greenapple R, Ngai J. Obesity: effective treatment requires change in payers' perspective. Am Health Drug Benefits 2010;3(2):88–94.
32. Kyle TK, Dhurandhar EJ, Allison DB. Regarding obesity as a disease: evolving policies and their implications. Endocrinol Metab Clin North Am 2016;45(3): 511–20.
33. Baum C, Andino K, Wittbrodt E, et al. The challenges and opportunities associated with reimbursement for obesity pharmacotherapy in the USA. Pharmacoeconomics 2015;33(7):643–53.
34. Espeland MA, Glick HA, Bertoni A, et al. Impact of an intensive lifestyle intervention on use and cost of medical services among overweight and obese adults with type 2 diabetes: the action for health in diabetes. Diabetes Care 2014; 37(9):2548–56.
35. MMIT formulary search for desktops. Available at: https://info.mmitnetwork.com/formulary. Accessed May 27, 2019.
36. Gomez G, Stanford FC. US health policy and prescription drug coverage of FDA-approved medications for the treatment of obesity. Int J Obes 2018;42(3): 495–500.
37. Doyle S, Lloyd A, Birt J, et al. Willingness to pay for obesity pharmacotherapy. Obesity 2012;20:2019–26.
38. O'Neil PM, Birkenfeld AL, McGowan B, et al. Efficacy and safety of semaglutide compared with liraglutide and placebo for weight loss in patients with obesity: a randomised, double-blind, placebo and active controlled, dose-ranging, phase 2 trial. Lancet 2018;392(10148):637–49.
39. Killion EA, Wang J, Yie J, et al. Anti-obesity effects of GIPR antagonists alone and in combination with GLP-1R agonists in preclinical models. Sci Transl Med 2018; 10(472):1–11.
40. Coskun T, Sloop KW, Loghin C, et al. LY3298176, a novel dual GIP and GLP-1 receptor agonist for the treatment of type 2 diabetes mellitus: from discovery to clinical proof of concept. Mol Metab 2018;18:3–14.
41. Number of ABOM diplomates tops 3,370 in US and Canada. American Board of Obesity Medicine Web site. Available at: https://www.abom.org/abom-adds-726/. Accessed August 2, 2019.

Endoscopic Treatments for Obesity

The Good, the Bad, and the Ugly

Aoife M. Egan, MB, PhD, Adrian Vella, MD*

KEYWORDS

- Endoscopy • Bariatric • Obesity • Intragastric balloon • Sleeve gastroplasty

KEY POINTS

- Bariatric surgery is an effective but invasive treatment for obesity, and medical therapies are frequently unsuccessful.
- Endoscopic approaches to obesity aim to provide an alternative option to traditional medical and surgical therapies.
- Gastric and small bowel endoscopic interventions may be associated with a significant short-term weight loss.
- Data on weight loss maintenance, long-term safety, and the role of endoscopic therapies in conjunction with other treatment modalities are lacking.
- Therefore, the risk/benefit ratio of such interventions is uncertain.

INTRODUCTION

The obesity epidemic began in most high-income countries in the 1970s and 1980s and is now affecting the majority of middle-income and many low-income countries.[1] Data from the National Health and Nutrition Examination Survey reveal that more than one-third of adults in the United States are obese (34.9%; 95% confidence interval [CI], 32.0%–37.9%) and more than two-thirds are either overweight or obese (68.5%; 95% CI, 65.2%–71.6%).[2] Consequently, there has been an increase in comorbidities related to obesity and it is estimated that the annual national medical care costs of obesity-related illness is $209.7 billion or 20.6% of United States' national health expenditures.[3]

Available treatments for weight loss include lifestyle interventions, pharmacotherapy, and bariatric surgery. Lifestyle interventions are associated with a modest initial weight loss, but the majority of people are unable to sustain the behaviors necessary to

Division of Endocrinology and Diabetes, Department of Medicine, Mayo Clinic, 200 First Street Southwest, Rochester, MN 55905, USA
* Corresponding author.
E-mail address: vella.adrian@mayo.edu

Endocrinol Metab Clin N Am 49 (2020) 315–328
https://doi.org/10.1016/j.ecl.2020.02.001

maintain weight loss.[4] For example, 811 overweight adults included in a randomized controlled trial of 4 dietary interventions lost an average of 7% of their initial weight at 6 months and began to regain weight after 12 months.[5] Weight loss medications are associated with a 5% to 10% loss in total body weight, but side effects are common and the long-term safety and efficacy is unclear.[6,7] In contrast, more than 50% weight loss is frequently achieved with bariatric surgery; however, less than 2% of eligible individuals receive these procedures.[8,9] It is likely that patient preference, cost, and associated morbidity and mortality are contributing to this treatment gap.[10]

Bearing this in mind, there is clearly a need for minimally invasive, safe, and effective interventions to treat obesity.[11] Endoscopic bariatric therapies have been developed as an alternative approach to noninvasive and surgical therapies, and multiple options are being evaluated or are available for clinical use. Moving forward, these treatments have the potential to play a major role in the obesity management algorithm in conjunction with other weight loss approaches. The aim of this review is to provide a comprehensive overview of endoscopic treatments for obesity, including their mechanisms of action, as well as their efficacy and safety.

ENDOSCOPIC BARIATRIC TREATMENTS: OVERVIEW

Endoscopic bariatric therapies may be divided into gastric and small bowel procedures (**Fig. 1**), each of which variably mimic at least some of the anatomic alterations created by bariatric surgery.[12] In this article, we address the established and emerging therapies and summarize the results of relevant clinical studies. Although the majority of studies refer to percent total weight loss, percent excess weight loss is also commonly reported. This latter metric depends on 3 variables, including the preprocedure weight, the postprocedure weight, and the ideal body weight. Because there are various definitions of ideal body weight, and the preprocedure period can last months (often with various dietary approaches during that timeframe), percent excess weight loss is prone to significant variance. One should therefore keep this variation in mind and take a cautious approach when interpreting results.[13] It is also important to appreciate that mere participation in clinical trials of a weight loss intervention is associated with significant weight loss. Therefore, intervention studies without a sham or placebo intervention need to be interpreted with caution.

GASTRIC ENDOSCOPIC BARIATRIC TREATMENTS

A decrease in gastric volume is a key component of bariatric surgical procedures. In addition to simply decreasing the gastric reservoir, it increases stimulation of gastric receptors and, in association with the decreased nutrient intake, results in alternation of orexigenic hormones.[14–17] By decreasing the compliance and volume of the stomach, such procedures may accelerate gastric emptying with increased secretion of duodenal hormones that may increase satiety.[18] Endoscopic therapies aim to achieve a similar effect by occupying space in the stomach, remodeling the stomach, or diverting nutrients away from the stomach. It should be noted that many of the trials place patients on an extremely restricted diet for the initial part of the study to protect the intervention. Caloric restriction per se can have important effects on diabetes and weight loss, again supporting the benefit of a sham arm subjected to the same dietary intervention when assessing results.[19,20]

Intragastric Balloons

The first intragastric balloon (IGB), the Garren-Edwards Gastric Bubble (American Edwards Laboratories, Irvine, CA), was actually approved in the United States in

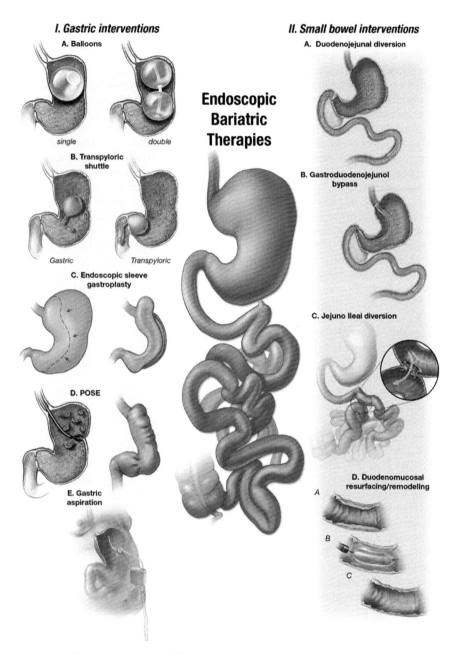

Fig. 1. Available gastric and small bowel interventions. (*From* Abu Dayyeh BK, Edmundowicz S, Thompson CC. Clinical practice update: Expert review on endoscopic bariatric therapies. Gastroenterology 2017;152(4):716-29; used with permission of Mayo Foundation for Medical Education and Research, all rights reserved.)

1985. This was an endoscopically placed, air-filled device. Unfortunately, it was poorly tolerated with numerous adverse events, including mucosal injury, and was eventually removed from the market when a randomized controlled trial failed to show any benefit compared with a sham insertion.[21] More recently, 3 IGBs have been approved by the US Food and Drug Administration for the treatment of obesity. All 3 devices are approved for 6 months of use.[12]

The Orbera IGB (Apollo Endosurgery, Austin, TX) was previously known as the Bio-Enterics Intragastric Balloon (Allergan, Irvine, CA) was actually developed in the early 1990s and has been used extensively outside of the United States.[4] It is a double-bagged polymer balloon covered with silicone that must be filled with air to a final volume of 650 to 750 mL. It is endoscopically implanted and removed. A systematic review and meta-analysis published in 2008 evaluated its safety and effectiveness for obesity.[22] This study included 15 articles and 3608 patients. The estimates for weight loss at balloon removal (6 months) were 14.7 kg or 12.2% of initial weight and 32.1% of excess weight. The majority of complications were mild and the early removal rate was low at 4.2%. Major complications were rare; for example, gastric perforation was noted in 0.1% and bowel obstruction in 0.8%. Although data on the long-term effectiveness are scant, 1 multicenter European study reported a mean excess weight loss of 55.6% at 6 months and 29.1% at 3 years.[23] There also seemed to be an association with balloon placement and a reduction in diabetes-related complications, with diabetes (defined as a fasting glycemia of $\geq$110 mg/dL and glycated hemoglobin of $\geq$6.0%) decreased from 15% to 10% from baseline to 3 years and hypertension decreased from 29% to 16%. In the United States, a multicenter, open-label, clinical trial randomized 255 adults with a body mass index (BMI) of 30 to 40 kg/m^2 to lifestyle intervention with or without the IGB.[24] At 9 months, the mean excess weight loss was 26.5% in the IGB and 9.7% in the control groups (P = .32). The majority of participants randomized to the IGB experienced gastrointestinal side effects and 18.8% had the IGB removed early owing to side effects or patient request.

The ReShape Duo IGB (Reshape, San Clemente, CA) is also endoscopically placed and retrieved and has 2 balloons attached to each other by a flexible tube. The balloons are each filled with 450 mL of a saline-methylene blue solution and the balloons have independent channels to prevent deflation of the other balloon if one leaks. The REDUCE trial (United States) randomized 326 participants with a BMI of 30 to 40 kg/m^2 to IGB plus diet and exercise or sham endoscopy plus diet and exercise. The intention-to-treat analysis revealed that IGB participants had a significantly greater percent excess weight loss at 24 weeks (25.1% vs 11.3%; P = .004).[25] In this trial, early retrieval was necessary in 15% participants. Although gastric ulcers and erosions were observed in more than one-third of participants, a minor device modification during the trial decreased this to 10.3%.

Finally, the Obalon IGB (Obalon Therapeutics, Carlsbsd, CA) is a 250-mL gas-filled balloon that is enclosed in a capsule attached to a slender tube that is swallowed under fluoroscopic visualization. If tolerated, a second balloon can be swallowed at 4 weeks and a third at 8 weeks. The balloons are removed endoscopically at 12 or 24 weeks.[4] A double-blind, randomized, sham-controlled trial of this balloon system plus lifestyle therapy compared with lifestyle therapy alone at 6 months in 387 participants with a BMI of 30 to 40 kg/m^2 was conducted in 15 centers across the United States.[26] Total weight loss in treatment and control groups were 7.1 $\pm$ 5.3 kg and 3.6 $\pm$ 5.1 kg ($P<$.0001), respectively, giving a mean difference of 3.5 kg. Although the majority of participants experienced mild adverse events, just 1 participant experienced a balloon deflation and another participant developed a bleeding ulcer.

The Spatz Adjustable balloon (Spatz Medical, Great Neck, NY) is currently not available in the United States, but is approved for 12-month use elsewhere. Available data suggest a 19% weight loss or 45.7% excess weight loss, but additional trial data are awaited.[27] The Elipse procedureless balloon (Allurion, Natick, MA) is swallowed while attached to a thin delivery catheter that is then filled with 550 mL of filling fluid. The catheter is then removed and the balloon resides in the stomach for 4 months. At this point, a valve opens, the balloon empties, and the empty balloon is then excreted. Initial studies have demonstrated a 10% total body weight loss with improvement in metabolic parameters such as glycated hemoglobin, triglycerides, and blood pressure, but a pivotal trial is pending.[28]

Nonballoon Space-Occupying Devices

The TransPyloric Shuttle (TPS; BAROnova, Goleta, CA) is an endoscopically placed and retrieved device that consists of a large, spherical bulb connected to a smaller cylindrical bulb by a flexible tether. It is composed predominantly of silicone and, once in the stomach, it moves freely and is designed to self-position across the pylorus during peristalsis to decrease gastric outflow. Essentially, it is intended to form an intermittent obstruction to delay gastric emptying and induce early satiation. A feasibility study included 20 participants with a mean BMI of 36 kg/m^2 assigned to the device for 3 or 6 months.[29] Participants allocated to the device for 3 months had an average excess weight loss of 25.1% and average weight loss of 8.9%. The 6-month participants had an average excess weight loss of 41.0% and average weight loss of 14.5%. Early device removal occurred in 2 patients owing to symptomatic gastric ulcerations, which resolved after device removal. A 12-month multicenter randomized controlled trial was subsequently undertaken in the United States, which resulted in US Food and Drug Administration approval for the device.[30] The ENDObesity II Study included 270 participants with a BMI of 30 to 40 kg/m^2 who were randomized in a 2:1 ratio to TPS or sham control. The mean percent total body weight loss at 12 months was 9.5% (95% CI, 8.2–10.8) in the TPS Group compared with 2.8% (95% CI, 1.1–4.5) for the control group. Ten percent of participants required early device removal owing to an adverse event and gastroduodenal ulcers were endoscopically observed in 10.3% of TPS participants; none developed bleeding or perforation.

The Full Sense Bariatric Device (Baker, Foote, Kemmeter, Walburn LLC, Grand Rapids, MI) is also endoscopically placed and removed, and incorporates an esophageal component and a gastric disc connected by a support.[31] It is designed to induce satiety in the absence of food by placing pressure on the distal esophagus and cardia of the stomach. This device is not yet approved for use either within or outside the United States and there are no peer-reviewed data to support its efficacy.

Aspiration Therapy

The AspireAssist (Aspire Bariatrics, King of Prussia, PA) allows removal of a portion of a meal approximately 20 minutes after consumption. The system comprises an endoscopically placed percutaneous gastrostomy tube and an external device to facilitate draining about one-third of the calories consumed in a meal. Two weeks after the tube is placed, the external portion is shortened and a skin port is attached flush with the skin. A connector is attached to the skin port that opens the closed skin port valve. Gastric contents then spontaneously flow out of the stomach through the drain tube into a toilet bowl. Remaining food particles are flushed out of the stomach with the assistance of an attached water reservoir, which flushes boluses of tap water into the stomach.[32] In the first trial 207 participants with a BMI of 35 to 55 kg/m^2 were randomly assigned in a 2:1 ratio to treatment with AspireAssist plus lifestyle counseling or lifestyle counseling alone. At 52 weeks, participants in the AspireAssist group, on a modified intent-to-treat basis, had lost 31.5 ± 26.7% of their excess body weight (12.1 ± 9.6% total body weight), compared with the lifestyle group who lost 9.8 ± 15.5% of their excess body weight (3.5 ± 6.0% total body weight)

(P<.001).[32] Adverse events include stoma granulation tissue (40.5%), stoma infection (14.4%), and gastric ulceration (0.9%). On completion of the study, participants were permitted to continue up to a maximum of 5 years, providing they maintained at least 10% total weight loss.[33] Approximately 70% participants elected to continue with the device and 40 (69%) achieved at least 10% weight loss at 4 years or time of study withdrawal. On a per-protocol basis, patients experienced 14.2%, 15.3%, 16.6%, and 18.7% total weight loss at 1, 2, 3, and 4 years, respectively (P<.01 for all). This device is currently approved in the United States for patients with a BMI of 35 to 55 kg/m^2. Given the mechanism of action of this device, concern was raised about the risk of triggering worsening eating behaviors; however, this has not been observed in the trials to date.

Endoscopic Suturing Procedures

Endoscopic sleeve gastroplasty decreases gastric capacity by creating an endoscopic sleeve, thus mimicking to a certain extent the surgical sleeve gastrectomy. The procedure involves the placement of full thickness sutures through the gastric wall, extending from the prepyloric antrum to the gastroesophageal junction.[12] An endoscopic suturing device (Overstitch; Apollo Endosurgery) may be used to facilitate the procedure. In general, patients undergoing this procedure consume a significantly modified diet in the subsequent weeks, for example, 2 to 3 weeks of liquid protein shakes, followed by 2 weeks of a puréed diet, before transitioning to a regular diet.

After an initial pilot study demonstrating feasibility, additional groups have published their clinical experience.[34,35] A longer term study included 248 participants with a baseline BMI of 37.8 kg/m^2 and reported that, at 6 and 24 months, percent total body weight loss was 15.2% (95% CI, 14.2–16.3) and 18.6% (95% CI, 15.7–21.5), respectively.[36] Serious adverse events occurred in 2% of patients, including perigastric inflammatory fluid collections requiring drainage and antibiotics, an extragastric hemorrhage requiring blood transfusion, and 1 pneumoperitoneum and pneumothorax. A systematic review and meta-analysis extracted data from 8 cohort studies including 1772 patients who underwent endoscopic sleeve gastroplasty.[37] Weight loss was sustained at 12 and 18 to 24 months after the procedure with a total body weight loss of 16.5% (95% CI, 15.2–17.8) and 17.2% (95% CI, 14.6–19.7), respectively. A low rate of serious adverse events was noted.

Primary obesity surgery endoluminal is another suturing procedure that uses an incisionless operating platform (USGI Medical, San Clemente, CA) with 4 working channels to place transmural tissue anchor plications that reduce accommodation of the gastric fundus. Typically, 8 to 9 plications are placed in the gastric fundus bringing the apex down to the gastroesophageal junction with a further 3 to 4 plications placed in the distal body to reduce gastric emptying.[4] A pivotal multicenter trial in the United States (ESSENTIAL trial) included 332 participants with a BMI of 30 kg/m^2 or greater and less than 35 kg/m^2 with at least 1 nonsevere comorbid obesity-related condition (uncontrolled or drug-dependent hypertension, type 2 diabetes, or hyperlipidemia) or a BMI of 35 kg/m^2 or greater and less than 40 kg/m^2 with or without a nonsevere obesity-related comorbid condition.[38] Participants were randomized 2:1 to receive the active or sham procedure and both groups received lifestyle intervention. The 12-month results were mean total body weight loss of 4.95 ± 7.04% in the active group and 1.38 ± 5.58% in the sham. Procedure-related serious adverse events were 5%, including hepatic abscess, extragastric bleeding, nausea, and vomiting.

Gastric Bypass Revision

Increased gastrojejunal stoma diameter is a risk factor for weight regain after Roux-en-Y gastric bypass.[39] Owing to the risks associated with revision surgery, endoscopic suturing has been explored as an option for stomal revision for over a decade.[11,40] Endoscopic transoral outlet reduction (TORe) **(Fig. 2)** was examined in the setting of a randomized controlled trial where 77 patients with weight regain or inadequate loss after a Roux-en-Y gastric bypass and a gastrojejunostomy diameter of more than 2 cm were randomized to TORe or a sham procedure.[41] At 6 months, participants who underwent TORe had a significantly greater mean percentage weight loss from baseline (3.5%; 95% CI, 1.8%–5.3%) than controls (0.4%; 95% CI, 2.3% weight gain to 3.0% weight loss) ($P = .021$). A further meta-analysis of 330 patients reported a pooled weight loss at 12 months of 8.4 kg (95% CI, 6.5–10.3 kg).[42] A combined approach of TORe plus gastroplasty of the gastric pouch from the gastroesophageal junction to the gastrojejunal stoma has also been reported in 20 obese patients with mean % excess weight loss of 39% and 53% at 3 and 6 months.[43]

SMALL BOWEL ENDOSCOPIC BARIATRIC TREATMENTS

The small intestine plays a key role in nutrient absorption and contains hormone-secreting enteroendocrine cells. The aims of small bowel endoscopic bariatric treatments are to bypass the passage of nutrients through the small bowel and resurface the duodenal mucosa.[10] Incisionless anastomoses systems are in the earlier stages of development.

Endobarrier

The EndoBarrier (Endobarrier GI Dynamics, Lexington, MA) is a duodenojejunal bypass sleeve comprising an impermeable polymer line measuring 65 cm. It is packaged in a delivery capsule, which is placed endoscopically with the assistance of fluoroscopy. Once it reaches the duodenal bulb, the sleeve is advanced into the small bowel and the anchoring crown is deployed.[10] This device results in food bypassing

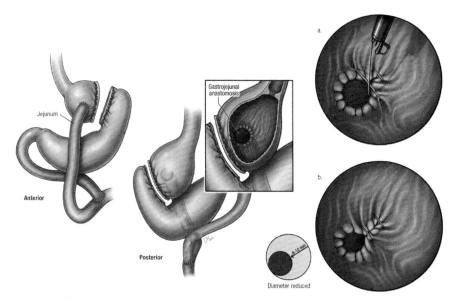

Fig. 2. An illustration of the endoscopic TORe procedure using a simple interrupted suture technique. The gastrojejunal diameter is decreased by 8 to 10 mm. Used with permission of Mayo Foundation for Medical Education and Research, all rights reserved.

the duodenum and proximal jejunum. It is removed endoscopically after 13 months. A systematic review and meta-analysis included 5 randomized controlled trials and 235 participants as well as 10 observational studies including 211 participants.[44] The mean BMI of the participants ranged from 30 to 49.2 kg/m^2. A meta-analysis showed that the duodenojejunal bypass sleeve was associated with significant mean differences in body weight and excess weight loss of −5.1 kg (95% CI, −7.3 to −3.0; 4 trials; n = 151; I^2 = 37%) and 12.6% (95% CI, 9.0–16.2; 4 trials; n = 166; I^2 = 24%), respectively, compared with diet modification. A multicenter double-blinded sham controlled trial in the United States was terminated early owing to a 3.5% incidence of hepatic abscess formation and, among those enrolled, early device retrieval owing to adverse events such as obstruction by a food bolus occurred in 11% patients.[10] Work is ongoing to develop modified devices with alternative anchoring mechanisms.

Endoluminal Bypass

The Endoluminal Bypass (Valen Tx, Maple Grove, MN) is a 120-cm liner endoscopically placed from the gastroesophageal junction to the small bowel. Its attachment is performed with 8 nitinol suture anchors that are deployed circumferentially and endoscopically ligated at study end.[45] It aims to mimic the Roux-en-Y gastric bypass and ideally remains in place for 12 months. This gastroduodenojejunal bypass sleeve was studied in 12 patients with a mean BMI of 42 kg/m^2.[45] Two patients were unable to tolerate the device, 4 were noted to have a partial cuff detachment at follow-up endoscopy, and 6 reached 1 year with a fully attached device. The latter 6 patients achieved a 54% excess weight loss and 5 of them were followed for an average of 14 months after explant and were found to have an average excess weight loss of 30%. Bowel erosions, ulceration, or pancreatitis were not reported and further trials are underway.

Duodenal Mucosal Resurfacing

Duodenal mucosal resurfacing (Fractyl, Lexington, MA) involves hydrothermal ablation of the duodenal mucosa via an endoscopic approach. The idea was developed in response to suggestions that bariatric bypass procedures produce weight loss and metabolic improvements that cannot be explained by a malabsorptive process alone.[46] Duodenal mucosal resurfacing therefore aims to alter the duodenal mucosal surface and manipulate downstream hormonal signaling. Most studies to date have included participants with type 2 diabetes with the intent of improving glycemic control.[47,48] One such international multicenter study included 46 participants with a BMI of 24 to 40 mg/m^2, of whom 38 underwent duodenal mucosal resurfacing.[47] Participants were fed a progressive diet moving from liquids to pureed foods to soft foods over 2 weeks. Glycated hemoglobin (−10 ± 2 mmol/mol [−0.9% ± 0.2%]; P<.001), fasting plasma glucose (−1.7 ± 0.5 mmol/L; P<.001), and Homeostatic Model Assessment of Insulin Resistance improved (−2.9 ± 1.1; P<.001), weight was modestly reduced (−2.5 ± 0.6 kg; P<.001), and hepatic transaminase levels decreased. These effects were sustained at 12 months.

Incisionless Magnetic Anastomotic System

The Incisionless Magnetic Anastomotic System (GI Windows, West Bridgewater, MA) uses self-assembling magnets to create an anastomosis with the aim of mimicking the duodenal switch and ileal transposition.[10] A compression anastomosis is formed after a week and the coupled magnets spontaneously pass. Both upper and lower endoscopy are required for placement. This system is still in the preliminary stages of development with data on 10 participants revealing a 14.6% (range, 0.3%–41.8%) total body weight loss at 1 year.[49]

DISCUSSION

In recognizing the magnitude and impact of obesity, we must also acknowledge the need for a paradigm shift in obesity management. Obese adults are typically faced with the option of bariatric surgery, which is invasive, costly, and typically reserved for individuals with severe obesity; or lifestyle modification and medical therapies, which are modestly effective and associated with significant recidivism.[50] As outlined, several endoscopic options for weight loss are now approved and available in the United States, with many more in the latter stages of development. Most of these therapies are indicated for patients with a BMI of 30 to 40 kg/m^2 who have been unable to achieve and sustain a weight loss with pharmacologic and/or lifestyle approaches.[10] Endoscopic procedures have the potential to change the treatment landscape and may provide an option for weight management that is less expensive and invasive than bariatric surgery. Although it is difficult to draw comparisons owing to the heterogeneity of the procedures and clinical trials, it seems that endoscopic procedures are more efficacious than currently available pharmacologic agents or lifestyle programs. For example, at 6 months the Orbera IGB is associated with a 12.2% loss of initial weight,[22] and the endoscopic sleeve gastrectomy is associated with an 18.6% loss of initial weight at 24 months.[36] This compares favorably with the 8.6% weight loss observed at 1 year in the intervention arm of the Look AHEAD study, a large randomized controlled trial of an intensive lifestyle intervention in overweight or obese adults with type 2 diabetes.[51] These endoscopic procedures also compare well with the 1-year pivotal trials of available weight loss medications, which are associated with a 5.8% to 9.8% loss of initial body weight.[52]

Worldwide, thousands of patients have received an IGB and their ease of insertion and reversibility makes them an attractive option.[53,54] However, data on long-term weight maintenance are lacking and one would anticipate significant weight regain after removal. A retrospective study reported greater weight loss with IGB therapy plus liraglutide (a glucagon-like peptide 1 agonist), but the combination did not seem to decrease the risk of weight regain after balloon removal.[55] Further high-quality studies assessing their use in tandem or sequentially with other treatment modalities would therefore be welcomed. It should also be noted that there are many situations where IGB placement is not suitable. For example, these devices are contraindicated in those with most upper gastrointestinal pathologies, coagulopathies, or in patients with an inability to use a proton pump inhibitor (**Box 1**).[56]

Likewise, although published studies of endoscopic plication procedures suggest excellent short-term weight loss, their long-term durability remains under question. Although the endoscopic sleeve gastroplasty is now widely practiced, there are no randomized controlled trials supporting its efficacy. Future research should examine its performance against lifestyle interventions and conventional bariatric procedures, such as laparoscopic sleeve gastrectomy.[37] Finally, although the drive to develop novel therapeutic approaches to metabolic conditions must be applauded, the acceptability and tolerability of any such strategies must be considered in detail. As an example, duodenal mucosal resurfacing procedures have the potential to cause duodenal stenosis and, given the likely need for repeat procedures, it is unlikely to be chosen over conventional therapies for type 2 diabetes.[46]

The upper gastrointestinal tract serves to assimilate ingested calories with hormonal, mechanical, and neural mechanisms and is instrumental in regulating postprandial glucose excursions.[18,57] To fully understand its mechanisms of action and anticipate medium and long-term outcomes, further studies should examine key physiologic pathways before and after endoscopic interventions and compare them with

---

Box 1
Contraindications for IGB therapy

Prior weight loss surgery or gastric surgery

Pregnancy or breast feeding

Alcoholism or drug abuse

Potential upper gastrointestinal bleeding conditions such as esophageal and gastric varices, arteriovenous malformations, or telangiectasias

Requirement for anticoagulation, aspirin, nonsteroidal anti-inflammatory drugs, or other gastric irritant

Large hiatal hernia greater than 5 cm, or less than 5 cm with associated severe gastroesophageal reflux disease symptoms

Any inflammatory disease of the gastrointestinal tract (esophagitis, gastritis, gastric or duodenal ulcers, cancer, or Crohn's disease)

Serious or uncontrolled psychiatric illness that may compromise the patient's compliance with balloon removal

Inability to tolerate endoscopy

Inability to take a proton pump inhibitor

Structural abnormality in the esophagus or pharynx, such as a stricture, that would impede the passage of the delivery catheter or endoscope

Gastric mass

Severe motility disorder that may pose a safety risk during balloon removal

Coagulopathy

Cirrhosis or hepatic insufficiency

Unwillingness to participate in a medically supervised weight loss program

Allergy to the material in the system

Patients with a history of serotonin syndrome and are currently taking a drug known to affect levels of serotonin in the body (if methylene blue is used in the balloon)

From Laing P, Pham T, Taylor LJ, Fang J. Filling the void: A review of intragastric balloons for obesity. Dig Dis Sci. 2017;62(6):1399-1408; with permission.

---

observation in individuals who undergo bariatric surgery and lifestyle programs. Indeed, it may be argued that, in many instances, investigators have not fully excluded the possibility that observed metabolic changes may be due to caloric restriction with a certain amount of sustained weight loss, rather than a predominant effect of the endoscopic procedure itself.[46] In support of this theory is prior work demonstrating that 6 weeks of caloric restriction to the levels typically used after bariatric surgery decreases fasting glucose and endogenous glucose production with improvements in beta cell function in people with type 2 diabetes.[19] With this information in mind, it is difficult to accept the alternative proposal that participants with type 2 diabetes secrete an unidentified factor from their proximal intestine that leads to insulin resistance and may be attenuated by bariatric procedures.[48]

SUMMARY

Endoscopic bariatric therapies is growing rapidly and has the potential to transform our approach to obesity management. Although long-term data are limited, short-term studies are promising and percent weight loss between that of pharmacologic and surgical interventions is expected. Emerging therapies should be evaluated rigorously before they are integrated into the multidisciplinary management of obesity. Beyond weight loss alone, we await randomized trials examining the effect of endoscopic procedures on metabolic parameters and other obesity-related comorbidities.

DISCLOSURE

Dr A. Vella receives funding from the National Institutes of Health (Grand IDs: DK78646, DK116231). Dr A.M. Egan has nothing to disclose.

REFERENCES

1. Swinburn BA, Sacks G, Hall KD, et al. The global obesity pandemic: shaped by global drivers and local environments. Lancet 2011;378(9793):804–14.
2. Ogden CL, Carroll MD, Kit BK, et al. Prevalence of childhood and adult obesity in the united states, 2011-2012. JAMA 2014;311(8):806–14.
3. Cawley J, Meyerhoefer C. The medical care costs of obesity: an instrumental variables approach. J Health Econ 2012;31(1):219–30.
4. Jirapinyo P, Thompson CC. Endoscopic bariatric and metabolic therapies: surgical analogues and mechanisms of action. Clin Gastroenterol Hepatol 2017;15(5): 619–30.
5. Sacks FM, Bray GA, Carey VJ, et al. Comparison of weight-loss diets with different compositions of fat, protein, and carbohydrates. N Engl J Med 2009; 360(9):859–73.
6. Kumar RB, Aronne LJ. Efficacy comparison of medications approved for chronic weight management. Obesity (Silver Spring) 2015;23(Suppl 1):S4–7.
7. Siebenhofer A, Jeitler K, Horvath K, et al. Long-term effects of weight-reducing drugs in people with hypertension. Cochrane Database Syst Rev 2016;(3):CD007654.
8. Buchwald H, Estok R, Fahrbach K, et al. Weight and type 2 diabetes after bariatric surgery: systematic review and meta-analysis. Am J Med 2009;122(3): 248–56.e5.
9. Sjoholm K, Anveden A, Peltonen M, et al. Evaluation of current eligibility criteria for bariatric surgery: diabetes prevention and risk factor changes in the Swedish Obese Subjects (SOS) study. Diabetes Care 2013;36(5):1335–40.
10. Vargas EJ, Rizk M, Bazerbachi F, et al. Medical devices for obesity treatment: endoscopic bariatric therapies. Med Clin North Am 2018;102(1):149–63.
11. Goyal D, Watson RR. Endoscopic bariatric therapies. Curr Gastroenterol Rep 2016;18(6):26.
12. Abu Dayyeh BK, Edmundowicz S, Thompson CC. Clinical practice update: expert review on endoscopic bariatric therapies. Gastroenterology 2017;152(4): 716–29.
13. Montero PN, Stefanidis D, Norton HJ, et al. Reported excess weight loss after bariatric surgery could vary significantly depending on calculation method: a plea for standardization. Surg Obes Relat Dis 2011;7(4):531–4.
14. Peterli R, Steinert RE, Woelnerhanssen B, et al. Metabolic and hormonal changes after laparoscopic Roux-en-Y gastric bypass and sleeve gastrectomy: a randomized, prospective trial. Obes Surg 2012;22(5):740–8.
15. Yousseif A, Emmanuel J, Karra E, et al. Differential effects of laparoscopic sleeve gastrectomy and laparoscopic gastric bypass on appetite, circulating acyl-

ghrelin, peptide yy3-36 and active glp-1 levels in non-diabetic humans. Obes Surg 2014;24(2):241–52.

16. Shah M, Laurenti MC, Dalla Man C, et al. Contribution of endogenous glucagon-like peptide-1 to changes in glucose metabolism and islet function in people with type 2 diabetes four weeks after Roux-en-Y gastric bypass (RYGB). Metabolism 2019;93:10–7.

17. Shah M, Law JH, Micheletto F, et al. Contribution of endogenous glucagon-like peptide 1 to glucose metabolism after Roux-en-Y gastric bypass. Diabetes 2014;63(2):483–93.

18. Ma J, Vella A. What has bariatric surgery taught us about the role of the upper gastrointestinal tract in the regulation of postprandial glucose metabolism? Front Endocrinol (Lausanne) 2018;9:324.

19. Sathananthan M, Shah M, Edens KL, et al. Six and 12 weeks of caloric restriction increases beta cell function and lowers fasting and postprandial glucose concentrations in people with type 2 diabetes. J Nutr 2015;145(9):2046–51.

20. Kelley DE, Wing R, Buonocore C, et al. Relative effects of calorie restriction and weight loss in noninsulin-dependent diabetes mellitus. J Clin Endocrinol Metab 1993;77(5):1287–93.

21. Hogan RB, Johnston JH, Long BW, et al. A double-blind, randomized, sham-controlled trial of the gastric bubble for obesity. Gastrointest Endosc 1989; 35(5):381–5.

22. Imaz I, Martinez-Cervell C, Garcia-Alvarez EE, et al. Safety and effectiveness of the intragastric balloon for obesity. A meta-analysis. Obes Surg 2008;18(7): 841–6.

23. Genco A, Lopez-Nava G, Wahlen C, et al. Multi-centre European experience with intragastric balloon in overweight populations: 13 years of experience. Obes Surg 2013;23(4):515–21.

24. Courcoulas A, Abu Dayyeh BK, Eaton L, et al. Intragastric balloon as an adjunct to lifestyle intervention: a randomized controlled trial. Int J Obes (Lond) 2017; 41(3):427–33.

25. Ponce J, Woodman G, Swain J, et al. The reduce pivotal trial: a prospective, randomized controlled pivotal trial of a dual intragastric balloon for the treatment of obesity. Surg Obes Relat Dis 2015;11(4):874–81.

26. Sullivan S, Swain J, Woodman G, et al. Randomized sham-controlled trial of the 6-month swallowable gas-filled intragastric balloon system for weight loss. Surg Obes Relat Dis 2018;14(12):1876–89.

27. Brooks J, Srivastava ED, Mathus-Vliegen EM. One-year adjustable intragastric balloons: results in 73 consecutive patients in the U.K. Obes Surg 2014;24(5): 813–9.

28. Machytka E, Gaur S, Chuttani R, et al. Elipse, the first procedureless gastric balloon for weight loss: a prospective, observational, open-label, multicenter study. Endoscopy 2017;49(2):154–60.

29. Marinos G, Eliades C, Raman Muthusamy V, et al. Weight loss and improved quality of life with a nonsurgical endoscopic treatment for obesity: clinical results from a 3- and 6-month study. Surg Obes Relat Dis 2014;10(5):929–34.

30. Weight reduction in patients with obesity using the Transpyloric Shuttle®:Endobesity® ii study. 2019. Available at: https://2018.obesityweek. com/abstract/weight-reduction-in-patients-with-obesity-using-the-transpyloric-shuttleendobesity-ii-study/. Accessed November 1, 2019

31. BFKW, LLC. Full Sense Device. Available at: http://www.bfkw.org/Home_Page. html. Accessed August 31, 2019.

32. Thompson CC, Abu Dayyeh BK, Kushner R, et al. Percutaneous gastrostomy device for the treatment of class ii and class iii obesity: results of a randomized controlled trial. Am J Gastroenterol 2017;112(3):447–57.

33. Thompson CC, Abu Dayyeh BK, Kushnir V, et al. Aspiration therapy for the treatment of obesity: 4-year results of a multicenter randomized controlled trial. Surg Obes Relat Dis 2019. https://doi.org/10.1016/j.soard.2019.04.026.

34. Abu Dayyeh BK, Rajan E, Gostout CJ. Endoscopic sleeve gastroplasty: a potential endoscopic alternative to surgical sleeve gastrectomy for treatment of obesity. Gastrointest Endosc 2013;78(3):530–5.

35. Kumar N, Abu Dayyeh BK, Lopez-Nava Breviere G, et al. Endoscopic sutured gastroplasty: procedure evolution from first-in-man cases through current technique. Surg Endosc 2018;32(4):2159–64.

36. Lopez-Nava G, Sharaiha RZ, Vargas EJ, et al. Endoscopic sleeve gastroplasty for obesity: a multicenter study of 248 patients with 24 months follow-up. Obes Surg 2017;27(10):2649–55.

37. Hedjoudje A, Dayyeh BA, Cheskin LJ, et al. Efficacy and safety of endoscopic sleeve gastroplasty: a systematic review and meta-analysis. Clin Gastroenterol Hepatol 2019. https://doi.org/10.1016/j.cgh.2019.08.022.

38. Sullivan S, Swain JM, Woodman G, et al. Randomized sham-controlled trial evaluating efficacy and safety of endoscopic gastric plication for primary obesity: the essential trial. Obesity (Silver Spring) 2017;25(2):294–301.

39. Abu Dayyeh BK, Lautz DB, Thompson CC. Gastrojejunal stoma diameter predicts weight regain after Roux-en-Y gastric bypass. Clin Gastroenterol Hepatol 2011; 9(3):228–33.

40. Thompson CC, Slattery J, Bundga ME, et al. Peroral endoscopic reduction of dilated gastrojejunal anastomosis after Roux-en-Y gastric bypass: a possible new option for patients with weight regain. Surg Endosc 2006;20(11):1744–8.

41. Thompson CC, Chand B, Chen YK, et al. Endoscopic suturing for transoral outlet reduction increases weight loss after Roux-en-Y gastric bypass surgery. Gastroenterology 2013;145(1):129–37.e3.

42. Vargas EJ, Bazerbachi F, Rizk M, et al. Transoral outlet reduction with full thickness endoscopic suturing for weight regain after gastric bypass: a large multicenter international experience and meta-analysis. Surg Endosc 2018;32(1): 252–9.

43. Goyal D, Kim S, Dutson E, et al. Endoscopic trans-oral outlet reduction in combination with gastroplasty (TORE-G) is a novel technique that is highly efficacious and safe for weight loss in patients with failed Roux-en-Y gastric bypass. Poster 186. Paper presented at: American College of Gastroenterology Annual Meeting 2015. Hawaii Convention Center Honolulu, Hawaii, USA, October 18, 2015.

44. Rohde U, Hedback N, Gluud LL, et al. Effect of the endobarrier gastrointestinal liner on obesity and type 2 diabetes: a systematic review and meta-analysis. Diabetes Obes Metab 2016;18(3):300–5.

45. Sandler BJ, Rumbaut R, Swain CP, et al. One-year human experience with a novel endoluminal, endoscopic gastric bypass sleeve for morbid obesity. Surg Endosc 2015;29(11):3298–303.

46. Garvey WT. Ablation of the duodenal mucosa as a strategy for glycemic control in type 2 diabetes: role of nutrient signaling or simple weight loss. Diabetes Care 2016;39(12):2108–10.

47. van Baar ACG, Holleman F, Crenier L, et al. Endoscopic duodenal mucosal resurfacing for the treatment of type 2 diabetes mellitus: one year results from the first

international, open-label, prospective, multicentre study. Gut 2019. https://doi.org/10.1136/gutjnl-2019-318349.

48. Rajagopalan H, Cherrington AD, Thompson CC, et al. Endoscopic duodenal mucosal resurfacing for the treatment of type 2 diabetes: 6-month interim analysis from the first-in-human proof-of-concept study. Diabetes Care 2016;39(12):2254–61.

49. Machytka E, Buzga M, Lautz DB, et al. 103: a dual-path enteral bypass procedure created by a novel incisionless anastomosis system (IAS): 6-months clinical results. Gastroenterology 2016;150(4):S26.

50. Khera R, Murad MH, Chandar AK, et al. Association of pharmacological treatments for obesity with weight loss and adverse events: a systematic review and meta-analysis. JAMA 2016;315(22):2424–34.

51. Look ARG, Wing RR, Bolin P, et al. Cardiovascular effects of intensive lifestyle intervention in type 2 diabetes. N Engl J Med 2013;369(2):145–54.

52. Heymsfield SB, Wadden TA. Mechanisms, pathophysiology, and management of obesity. N Engl J Med 2017;376(15):1492.

53. Saber AA, Shoar S, Almadani MW, et al. Efficacy of first-time intragastric balloon in weight loss: a systematic review and meta-analysis of randomized controlled trials. Obes Surg 2017;27(2):277–87.

54. Yorke E, Switzer NJ, Reso A, et al. Intragastric balloon for management of severe obesity: a systematic review. Obes Surg 2016;26(9):2248–54.

55. Mosli MM, Elyas M. Does combining liraglutide with intragastric balloon insertion improve sustained weight reduction? Saudi J Gastroenterol 2017;23(2):117–22.

56. Laing P, Pham T, Taylor LJ, et al. Filling the void: a review of intragastric balloons for obesity. Dig Dis Sci 2017;62(6):1399–408.

57. Vella A, Camilleri M. The gastrointestinal tract as an integrator of mechanical and hormonal response to nutrient ingestion. Diabetes 2017;66(11):2729–37.

Common and Rare Complications of Bariatric Surgery

Maria L. Collazo-Clavell, MD, Meera Shah, MBChB*

KEYWORDS

- Bariatric surgery • Complications • Nutritional deficiencies

KEY POINTS

- Nutritional deficiencies after bariatric surgery are related to anatomic changes that are specific to the surgery type.
- Multivitamin supplementation regimens following bariatric surgery should be tailored to surgical type and presence of preexisting nutritional deficiencies.
- There is a higher risk of nephrolithiasis following gastric bypass because of fat malabsorption.
- Post–gastric bypass hypoglycemia is a rare complication of gastric bypass surgery and often requires multiple modalities of treatment.
- Patients undergoing bariatric surgery should be screened for and counseled on the effects of alcohol use before and after surgery.

INTRODUCTION

An increasing number of individuals are choosing to undergo bariatric surgery as a result of its proven efficacy at promoting weight loss and improvement of many weight-related medical comorbidities.[1] However, bariatric operations can be associated with complications that can negatively affect health. The risk for these complications can be mitigated through active surveillance. The responsibility of surveillance often falls on the primary care provider because a large percentage of patients who have undergone bariatric surgery are lost to follow-up from their bariatric surgery programs.[2]

NUTRITIONAL DEFICIENCIES

Several factors contribute to the risk for nutrient deficiencies after bariatric surgery. A high percentage of patients seeking bariatric surgery have unrecognized nutrient

Division of Endocrinology, Diabetes and Nutrition, Mayo Clinic, 200 1st Street Southwest, Rochester, MN 55905, USA
* Corresponding author.
E-mail address: Shah.Meera@mayo.edu

Endocrinol Metab Clin N Am 49 (2020) 329–346
https://doi.org/10.1016/j.ecl.2020.02.003
0889-8529/20/© 2020 Elsevier Inc. All rights reserved.

deficiencies before any operation is performed. Despite the surplus of calories consumed, diets are low in foods of high nutritional value.[3,4]

Macronutrient (carbohydrate, protein, fats) deficiencies are rare. However, micronutrient deficiencies are not. Vitamin D deficiency is by far the most common, reported in up to 92% of bariatric surgery candidates. The risk of vitamin D deficiency is inversely related to body mass index (BMI) and is often associated with secondary hyperparathyroidism.[3]

Although prevalence rates vary among published studies, deficiencies in iron, calcium, vitamin B_{12}, folate, and vitamin B1 have also been reported among bariatric surgery candidates[3,4] (**Table 1**). As a result, current guidelines propose routine screening for commonly identified micronutrients and appropriate supplementation started.[4]

The risk for nutrient deficiencies is further influenced by which weight loss operation is performed. Gastric restrictive operations do not alter gut continuity and should not

Table 1
Prevalence of nutrient deficiencies, recommended nutrient supplementation, and recommended testing for patients undergoing bariatric surgery

Deficiencies	Preoperative Prevalence Rates	Postoperative SG Prevalence Rates	Postoperative RYGB Prevalence Rates	Postoperative BPD-DS Prevalence Rates
Vitamin D (<30 ng/mL) (<50 nmol/L)	71.7%–100% 81%	24.3%	Up to 100%	Up to 100%
Folate (<4.6 ng/mL) (<100 nmol/L)	0%–32% 8.4%–24%	—	Up to 65%	Up to 65%
Vitamin B_{12} (<350 pg/mL) (<150 pmol/L)	37% 8.4%–11.5%	4%–20%	<20%	52% at 10 y
Iron Ferritin Men <30 μg/L Women < 20 μg/L	7%	37.8% at 5 y	20%–55%	8%–50%
Vitamin B_1 (<32 pg/L) (<70 nmol/L)	6% 5.5%	Up to 49%*	—	—
Vitamin A <20 μg/L	1.7%	—	Up to 70%	Up to 70%
Zinc (<70 μg/dL) (<10 μmol/L)	2.9% 0.5%	19%	40%	Up to 70%
Copper (<70 μg/dL)	0%	Rare	10%–20%	Up to 90%
Calcium (<8.5 mg/dL)* (<2.2 mmol/L)	13.3% 13.7%	—	—	37.2% at 5 y
Protein (Albumin < 3.6 g/dL)	1.1%	4.2% at 5 y	—	50% at 10 y

(continued on next page)

Table 1 (continued)				
Deficiencies	Preoperative Prevalence Rates	Postoperative SG Prevalence Rates	Postoperative RYGB Prevalence Rates	Postoperative BPD-DS Prevalence Rates
Recommended nutritional supplementation	MVI/minerals 100% RDI Vitamin D	Vitamin B$_1$ 100%–200% RDI Folate >100% RDI Iron >100% RDI Vitamin B$_{12}$ Oral 350–500 μg/d SQ/IM 1000 μg/mo Vitamin D >3000 IU/d Calcium 1200–1500 mg/d Vitamin A 100%–200% RDI Copper and zinc 100% RDI	Vitamin B$_1$ 100%–200% RDI Folate 100%–200% RDI Iron 100%–200% RDI Vitamin B$_{12}$ Oral 350–500 μg/d SQ/IM 1000 μg/mo Vitamin D >3000 IU/d Calcium 1200–1500 mg/d Vitamin A 100%–200% RDI Copper and zinc 100%–200% RDI	Vitamin B$_1$ 100%–200% RDI Folate 100%–200% RDI Iron 100%–200% RDI Vitamin B$_{12}$ Oral 350–500 μg/d SQ/IM 1000 μg/mo Vitamin D >3000 IU/d Calcium 1800–2400 mg/d Vitamin A 10,000 IU/d Copper and zinc 200% RDI
Recommended testing	CBC, ferritin 25-OH vitamin D Folate Vitamin B$_{12}$ Thiamine Calcium*	CBC, ferritin Folate* Vitamin B$_{12}$ Vitamin D Thiamine**	CBC, ferritin Folate* Vitamin B$_{12}$* Vitamin D Vitamin A Copper Zinc Thiamine**	CBC, ferritin Folate Vitamin B$_{12}$ Vitamin D Vitamin A Copper Zinc Thiamine
—	—	—	24-h urine supersaturation	24-h urine supersaturation

* Laboratory result on routine supplementation.
** Laboratory result after supplementation adjustment.
  Abbreviations: BPD-DS, biliopancreatic diversion with duodenal switch; CBC, complete blood count; IM, intramuscular; MVI, multiple vitamins injection; RDI, recommended daily intake; RYGB, Roux en Y gastric bypass; SG, sleeve gastrectomy; SQ, subcutaneous.
  Data from Roust LR, DiBaise JK. Nutrient deficiencies prior to bariatric surgery. Curr Opin Clin Nutr Metab Care. 2017; 20(2):138-144 and Parrott J, Frank I, Rabena R, et al. American Society for Metabolic and Bariatric Surgery Integrated Health Nutritional Guidelines for the Surgical Weight Loss Patient 2016 Update: Micronutrients. Surg Obes Relat Dis. 2017; 13(5): 727-741.

impair nutrient absorption from an anatomic perspective (**Fig. 1**). However, nutrient deficiencies have been reported after solely gastric restrictive procedures, suggesting that other factors contribute. The most common deficiencies reported after sleeve gastrectomy (SG) are vitamin D, followed by iron and vitamin B$_{12}$.[4,5] Some of these deficiencies may have been preexisting.[3,4] However, the restrictive effect on food intake, the presence of gastrointestinal symptoms, and medications can further increase the

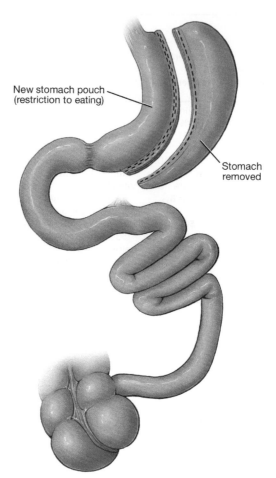

New stomach pouch
(restriction to eating)

Stomach
removed

Fig. 1. Sleeve gastrectomy. (Used with permission of Mayo Foundation for Medical Education and Research, all rights reserved.)

risk. Dietary intakes after gastric restrictive operations are lower in calories but also lower in nutrients with protein intakes of less than 60 g daily within the first 3 months after surgery.[6] Protein intakes gradually improve but remain significantly less than pre-operative intakes up to a year.[7] Most individuals seeking bariatric surgery are women of reproductive age who may already be at risk for iron deficiency.[8] Thiamin deficiency and Wernicke encephalopathy have been reported in patients with persistent vomiting after gastric restrictive operations. Liberation of cobalamin from foods requires an acid environment, and deficiencies in vitamin B_{12} can occur with the chronic use of proton pump inhibitors and/or the absence of gastric acid from a small gastric pouch.[4]

In addition to dietary restriction created by a small gastric pouch (30 cm³), the Roux en Y gastric bypass (RYGB) introduces a bypass of the distal stomach and duodenum (**Fig. 2**). The duodenum is the main intestinal site for iron and calcium absorption.[9] The Roux limb limits intraluminal interaction of biliary and pancreatic enzymes with food, introducing malabsorption of nutrients. In addition to deficiencies previously outlined, deficiencies in calcium, zinc, copper, and other fat-soluble vitamins, such as vitamin A, are more common after the RYGB.[4] Coexistence of multiple nutrient deficiencies is

Anatomy of Roux-en-Y

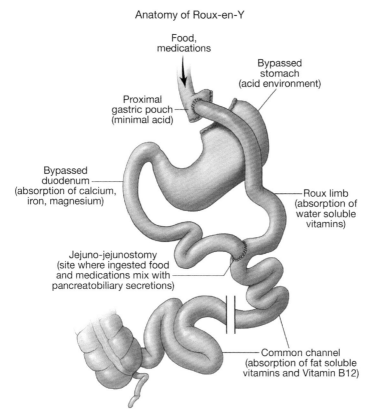

Fig. 2. RYGB. (Used with permission of Mayo Foundation for Medical Education and Research, all rights reserved.)

common. Iron deficiency may mask coexisting copper deficiency because both can present with microcytic anemias. In addition to anemia and leukopenia, severe copper deficiency can result in gait abnormalities and peripheral neuropathies, which, if untreated, can result in permanent disability. Severe zinc deficiency can result in diarrhea, listlessness, and eczematous lesions around the nasolabial folds, perioral skin, perineum, and scrotum. Hair loss and alopecia may also develop. Copper deficiency can coexist with zinc deficiency because they often result from excessive intestinal losses; for example, in patients with diarrhea. If not recognized, zinc supplementation can precipitate copper deficiency because absorption of these minerals is a competitive process.[4]

Operations that introduce fat malabsorption as the main mechanism for weight loss include the biliopancreatic diversion, the biliopancreatic diversion and duodenal switch, and the now-abandoned ileojejunal bypass. The biliopancreatic diversion and duodenal switch is currently the most common malabsorptive operation offered but the least commonly performed.[10] This operation involves the creation of an SG that introduces restriction with a duodenal switch preserving the pylorus and a bypass of the biliopancreatic limb with biliary and pancreatic juices entering the distal 100 cm of ileum, referred to as the common channel[11,12] (**Fig. 3**). The prevalence of nutrient deficiencies is higher and of greater severity than with operations previously discussed.[4,11,12] The coexistence of multiple nutrient deficiencies is common, including

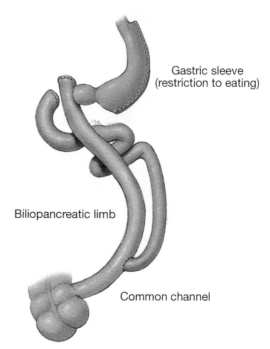

Gastric sleeve
(restriction to eating)

Biliopancreatic limb

Common channel

Fig. 3. Biliopancreatic diversion with duodenal switch. (Used with permission of Mayo Foundation for Medical Education and Research, all rights reserved.)

fat-soluble vitamins and mineral deficiencies despite active supplementation,[13] which makes long-term nutritional surveillance and active modification to supplementation regimens necessary to avoid deficiencies. Unlike gastric restrictive operations and the RYGB, the biliopancreatic diversion and duodenal switch can lead to macronutrient deficiency with protein malnutrition. Protein malnutrition is the most common indication for revision of this surgery at a rate of 5% per year.[11,12] As a result, modifications to this operation have been recommended by lengthening the common channel up to 200 cm. A recent report suggests this modification can reduce the risk for nutrient deficiencies but at the expense of long-term weight loss.[14]

The high prevalence of nutrient deficiencies after bariatric surgery has led to the implementation of empiric vitamin and mineral supplementation (see **Table 1**). Supplementation regimens vary among bariatric surgery programs, but recent guidelines are designed to introduce some structure to the regimens implemented. Multivitamin and mineral supplementation ideally should contain iron and provide 100% to 200% of recommended daily intake (RDI).[4] This supplementation has been shown to reduce the risk for deficiencies of folate, iron, copper, zinc, and selenium.[15,16] Additional supplementation of vitamin B_{12} is necessary. Both oral and parenteral supplementation are acceptable but ongoing surveillance of vitamin B_{12} levels is recommended with oral supplementation. If a patient is adherent to parenteral vitamin B_{12} supplementation, deficiency is rare and laboratory monitoring not necessary.[4,16] Current guidelines recommend vitamin D supplementation at 3000 international units (IU) daily.[4] However, higher doses may be required after RYGB or malabsorptive operations to achieve 25-OH vitamin D levels greater than 30 ng/mL, which are ideal for bone health.[17] Calcium supplementation needs are influenced by patient age, surgery performed, and post–bariatric surgery diet. For those individuals with limited intake of calcium-rich foods, calcium supplementation is necessary.[4] Monitoring calcium needs can be challenging because hypocalcemia is a late finding in calcium deficiency. Measurement of 24-hour urine calcium excretion can guide supplementation needs. A low urinary calcium excretion (excretion <50 mg per 24 hours) suggests the body is calcium depleted, a potential contributor to secondary hyperparathyroidism.[9] In our practice, we titrate calcium supplementation to achieve 24-hour urine calcium excretion of at least 100 to 200 mg per 24 hours.[16] Iron deficiency is common and studies have reported that empiric iron supplementation can reduce the risk.[16] However, additional iron supplementation may be necessary. As a result, monitoring for iron deficiency and identifying those individuals who need additional supplementation beyond that provided in multivitamin/mineral preparation are recommended.[4,16] Vitamin A deficiency is most commonly identified among patients who have undergone malabsorptive operations requiring additional supplementation. However, up to 25% of patients after RYGB develop vitamin A deficiency as well.[4]

Nutritional monitoring is recommended in patients seeking bariatric surgery and is continued after surgery. Type and frequency of monitoring can vary depending on the operation performed and empiric vitamin supplementation regimen recommended. Patient-related factors can also affect monitoring, such as adherence to supplementation advised and the development of health conditions that might affect nutrition. However, it is important that each program develops a protocol for standard supplementation and monitoring and educates patients regarding the importance of ongoing surveillance in order to minimize the risk for nutritional deficiencies that can affect their wellness.[4]

BONE LOSS

Given the high prevalence of deficiencies in vitamin D and calcium among individuals seeking bariatric surgery, it is not surprising that bone health may be at risk. Increased bone turnover and bone loss have been routinely observed after bariatric surgery.[18] However, an increased risk of fractures is only consistently reported after malabsorptive operations such as the biliopancreatic diversion. The types of fractures vary. Fractures of the distal lower limb are more common before surgery, whereas classic osteoporosis pattern fractures of the upper limb and spine are more prevalent after surgery.[19]

Several factors contribute to increased bone turnover and bone loss observed after bariatric surgery.[20] Physiologic adaptation from decreased mechanical loading on the skeleton has been observed even after modest weight loss.[21,22] The development of secondary hyperparathyroidism from deficiencies in vitamin D, calcium, or both can further affect bone loss.[23] Women, who more commonly undergo bariatric surgery than men, may also have the additional risk factor of estrogen deficiency as they enter menopause.[24] Other patient-related factors affecting bone metabolism can include immobility, medical comorbidities, and medications.

In order to protect bone health, reversible factors that contribute to bone loss must be addressed. These factors include changes in mechanical loading and nutrition. Ensuring adequate intake of protein, vitamin D, and calcium is of particular importance in this patient population. Several investigators have shown that optimizing intake of protein, calcium, and vitamin D can mitigate the increased bone turnover and bone loss observed after bariatric surgery.[22,25] Muschitz and colleagues[25] studied the impact of vitamin D, calcium, and protein loading with physical exercise among individuals scheduled to undergo either RYGB or SG. This study was a 24-month prospective intervention trial. The intervention cohort received 28,000 IU/wk of vitamin D for 8 weeks before surgery, followed by 16,000 IU of vitamin D weekly and 1000 mg of calcium daily after surgery. Bone turnover markers, vitamin D, parathyroid hormone, and bone mineral density were measured. Both cohorts were observed to have increased bone turnover markers highest at 6 months postsurgery. However, the intervention cohort experienced less severe increases in bone turnover markers and less significant decrease in bone mineral density measurements at the spine, hip, and total compared with standard practice. Hence, dietary interventions can have a beneficial impact on bone turnover and protect against excessive bone loss.

Recommended calcium intakes after bariatric surgery vary depending on operation performed[4] (see **Table 1**). However, increased bone turnover and bone loss can still occur despite recommended supplementation of calcium after RYGB.[9] Current guidelines for vitamin D supplementation after bariatric surgery recommend at least 3000 IU of vitamin D_3 daily.[4] However, higher supplementation is often necessary to achieve optimal 25-OH vitamin D levels more than 30 ng/mL.[16,17] No additional protein supplementation is advised beyond that recommended after bariatric surgery.[20]

Physical activity is strongly encouraged after bariatric surgery. Both aerobic and weight training exercises provide benefits at protecting lean muscle mass during weight loss. Both types of exercises when instituted soon after bariatric surgery have been associated with a lower increase in bone turnover markers and less decrease in bone mineral density at 1 year after RYGB. Although physical activity interventions varied, they have consistently included at least 120 minutes of exercise a week (120–180 min/wk) and at least 2 sessions of weight bearing and strength training per week.[25,26]

Protecting bone health after bariatric surgery involves several interventions: (1) ensuring adequate nutrition is achieved by both dietary intake and nutrient supplementation, (2) monitoring nutritional parameters to avoid deficiencies, and (3) encouraging regular physical activity that includes both aerobic and weight-bearing exercises. Measurement of bone turnover markers is not routinely recommended after bariatric surgery. Measurement of bone mineral density in the absence of an established diagnosis of osteoporosis is generally recommended 2 years after surgery when eating habits are established and nutrient supplementation optimized.[20]

NEPHROLITHIASIS

Obesity (BMI>30 kg/m^2) is a risk factor for kidney stone formation, most commonly uric acid stones associated with insulin resistance.[27,28] Weight loss after bariatric surgery does not mitigate the risk for kidney stone formation. On the contrary, several studies have reported a higher incidence of nephrolithiasis, mainly of calcium oxalate stones. The risk for nephrolithiasis is highest for malabsorptive surgeries such as jejunoileal bypass, which is no longer performed, and the biliopancreatic diversion and duodenal switch. Reported prevalence rates range from 22% to 28%. The RYGB carries a moderate risk, with prevalence rates of 7.65% to 13%.[28] Solely gastric restrictive operations are not associated with higher risk for kidney stone formation beyond that attributed to obesity.[28,29]

Several processes contribute to calcium oxalate stone formation. All bariatric operations restrict eating and drinking. As a result, urinary volumes decrease significantly after bariatric surgery, which is conducive to urinary crystal formation.[29–31] Surgeries that induce malabsorption of fatty acids lead to increased absorption of oxalate.

Under normal circumstances, intraluminal oxalate is usually bound by dietary calcium and excreted in the stool. In the presence of fat malabsorption, intraluminal calcium is bound to intraluminal fatty acids, rendering oxalate available for absorption. Oxalate absorption is further enhanced by increased mucosal permeability to oxalate promoted by bile acid malabsorption. The oxalate absorbed in the colon is excreted by the kidneys, leading to hyperoxaluria. Precipitation of calcium oxalate and calcium citrate in the urine is inhibited by urinary citrate. Hypocitraturia observed after RYGB represents another factor contributing to calcium oxalate crystallization.[29]

After RYGB, increases in urinary calcium oxalate supersaturation are observed as early as 2 months after surgery. Nephrolithiasis can present as early as the first year after surgery.[28,31,32] As a result, implementing interventions to prevent kidney stone formation and identifying the individuals at risk should be instituted soon after surgery.

After bariatric surgery, individuals can find it challenging to ingest the 1.9 L (64 ounces) of fluid a day recommended and patients should be strongly encouraged to track their intake of fluids. Frequent visits with a dietitian in the first year after surgery are the standard of care. Their role is critical in providing ongoing advice to help the patients meet nutrition and hydration goals. Dietitians can monitor dietary intake of macronutrients and micronutrients, particularly foods rich in calcium and oxalate, which can affect the risk for the development of kidney stones. Among patients who have undergone bariatric surgery, dietary calcium intake is often low. As a result, calcium supplementation is often recommended.[32–34]

Identifying the patients at risk for the development of calcium oxalate stones can be challenging. A 24-hour urine supersaturation study can provide valuable information. Although tedious for the patients to complete, results can identify whether the patient is drinking an adequate amount of fluids (by assessing total volume excretion), ingesting adequate calcium, has increased oxalate excretion, has low urinary citrate level, and increased risk for calcium oxalate crystallization. Identifying risk factors to kidney stone formation offers the opportunity to intervene. Current recommendations suggest completing a 24-hour urine supersaturation at 6 to 12 months after surgery. Test can be completed earlier, particularly in patients with a history of renal stone disease, but abnormalities observed may not be a good reflection of patient's long-term risk because dietary intake remains significantly restricted.[32,34]

Once a patient is identified as being at risk for calcium oxalate stones, the standard of care for treatment includes the following key elements: (1) adequate fluid intake (urine volumes >1500 mL per 24 hours or >2000 mL in those with known calcium oxalate stones); (2) low-fat diet; (3) low-oxalate diet (<100 mg/d); (4) replete dietary calcium (1200 mg/d); (5) use of supplemental calcium pills dosed with meals (up to 3 g elemental calcium per day); and (6) correction of hypocitraturia with potassium citrate salts.[28,29,32,34]

POST–GASTRIC BYPASS HYPOGLYCEMIA

Since publication of the first case series of patients experiencing hyperinsulinemic hypoglycemia following RYGB in 2005,[35] this unique phenomenon has become increasingly recognized in bariatric surgery patients.

Epidemiologic studies show that postprandial hypoglycemia following gastric bypass most commonly occurs after the first 1 to 2 years of surgery, and typically 1 to 3 hours after eating.[36,37] It is estimated that approximately 10% of patients who undergo gastric bypass develop significant hypoglycemia, with less than 1% developing severe hypoglycemia, defined as a blood glucose level of less than or equal to 40 mg/dL, and emergency room visit or hospitalization for hypoglycemia.[38] Symptoms of hypoglycemia can range from adrenergic manifestations (abdominal cramping, nausea, sweats, and diarrhea) to more serious neuroglycopenic sequelae. For some patients, symptoms are recurrent and recalcitrant, affecting functioning and overall quality of life. Interestingly, it has also been shown that hypoglycemia, as defined by continuous glucose monitoring of less than 55 mg/dL, occurred in approximately 70% of patients for a mean duration of 71 minutes (including overnight), although no symptom correlation was provided.[39] There is currently no predictive clinical tool to identifying at-risk patients.

Expert opinion is divergent in terms of how best to diagnose hypoglycemia after gastric bypass, with liquid mixed meals and solid mixed meals both used in research settings.[40,41] Ultimately, patients with post–gastric bypass hypoglycemia should be able to fulfill the Whipple triad (low venous glucose level, with symptoms, and improved with carbohydrate ingestion) to be given the diagnosis. Symptoms should not occur in the fasting state.

The pathophysiology of post–gastric bypass hypoglycemia seems to involve process-specific surgical changes, nutrient delivery, and enteroinsulin hormone axis activity. Patients who undergo RYGB have an altered anatomy that allows rapid transit of nutrients from the gastric pouch into the small bowel (Roux limb). Dumping syndrome, first described in patients undergoing gastroenterostomy a century ago, is a result of the rapid emptying of nutrients into the small bowel, leading to higher-osmolality contents in the small bowel.[42] The result is a cascade of hormonal changes that lead to vasomotor and gastrointestinal symptoms such as tachycardia and cramping.

The term delayed dumping has been interchangeably used with postprandial hypoglycemia, highlighting the importance of timing of symptoms in relation to a meal. Hypoglycemia occurs as a result of an exaggerated insulin response to food intake, driven by changes in the upper gastrointestinal tract. Following meal ingestion, there is an earlier peak glucose response accompanied by higher glucagonlike peptide 1 (GLP-1, an incretin) secretion, both of which drive hyperinsulinemia.[43,44] Experimental conditions that block the GLP-1 receptor postprandially can reduce insulin secretion and lessen hypoglycemia.[45] However, other factors, including the inappropriate persistence of hypoglycemia because of altered α-cell or β-cell function, and delayed clearance of insulin, are likely also contributory.[40] In addition, abnormal enteroinsular axis activity in affected individuals may contribute to the increased susceptibility to hypoglycemia, along with other insulin-independent processes.[46] In sum, postprandial hypoglycemia following gastric bypass surgery is a result of altered glucose delivery and use triggering hyperinsulinemia, against a backdrop of several altered pancreatic and enteral hormonal axes.

Treatment of postprandial hypoglycemia starts with a comprehensive review of the patient's dietary patterns and choices. Skilled bariatric dieticians are usually able to identify specific areas for change (eg, carbohydrate choice, speed of eating, liquid consumption with meals), which can reduce the severity and/or frequency of these episodes. In the absence of well-designed clinical studies to guide macronutrient quality, quantity, or timing, our general approach is to eliminate high-glycemic-index carbohydrates where possible and encourage protein and fat consumption with complex carbohydrates, in line with the recommendations provided by Suhl and colleagues.[47] We also emphasize the importance of avoiding alcohol and excessive caffeine consumption, both of which increase the risk of postprandial hypoglycemia by impairing hepatic glucose release. In our experience, about two-thirds of patients have adequate symptom relief with dietary modification alone. Adjunctive treatment with medications that slow the absorption of glucose (eg, acarbose) or reduce the secretion of insulin (eg, octreotide or diazoxide) may be considered but are limited by side effects and efficacy (**Table 2**). The GLP-1 receptor agonist liraglutide has been used for its ability to delay gastric emptying and therefore delivery of nutrients into the Roux limb. However, the quality of evidence supporting pharmacologic therapies is poor, and, in our clinical experience, response can be heterogenous.[48,49]

Procedural options short of gastric bypass reversal also exist and may be considered if other modalities are unsuccessful. Endoscopic plication of the gastrojejunal anastomosis serves to reduce the size of the gastric outlet and therefore slow down the rate of emptying of nutrients out of the pouch. In a small case series, patients reported improvement in symptoms 1 month following the procedure; however, what is unknown is the durability of these results, particularly once the patient has transitioned off the postprocedural diet.[50] The authors and others have used enteral feeding into the gastric remnant, which essentially serves to recruit the pylorus and proximal small bowel during feeding.[51] Some patients are able to tolerate bolus feeds, whereas others require continuous tube feeds to be symptom free. This approach clearly has an impact on quality of life and patients still have to restrict carbohydrate consumption by mouth. However, it is a reasonable option for patients who might otherwise be of high surgical risk and who are willing and able to administer tube feeds. Partial pancreatectomy is high risk and results in incomplete resolution of hypoglycemic episodes; it is therefore not a recommended treatment option.[52]

In summary, hypoglycemia after RYGB is an infrequent complication, and severe episodes are rare. However, management of symptoms can be challenging and may involve the use of several different treatment modalities. Patient counseling with regard to natural history and expectations is key.

Although there are reports of hypoglycemia following surgical SG, there are no reliable data on the prevalence of this condition.

Table 2
Pharmacotherapy options for the treatment of post–Roux-en-Y gastric bypass hypoglycemia

	Mechanism of Action	Studied Dose	Side Effects
Acarbose[76]	Delays and reduces absorption of glucose by inhibition of intestinal α-glucosidase	50 mg orally 4–5 times before meals	Bloating, cramps, excess abdominal gas
Diazoxide[77,78]	Reduces insulin secretion by inhibition of β-cell ATP-sensitive potassium channels	50–100 mg orally twice daily	Fluid retention, nausea, headache, hypotension, hirsutism
Octreotide[48]	Reduces insulin and GLP-1 secretion by binding to somatostatin receptors subtypes 2 and 5	25–50 μg subcutaneously before meals	Abdominal pain, nausea, diarrhea, headache, cholelithiasis
Liraglutide[49]	Delays gastric emptying; may reduce insulin secretion during low-glucose state	1.2–1.8 mg subcutaneously daily	Nausea, bloating

Data from Refs.[48,49,76–78]

ALCOHOL USE DISORDER

Anatomic changes that occur during gastric bypass surgery alter the pharmacokinetics of alcohol metabolism.[53,54] The rate of delivery of ingested alcohol into the systemic circulation is increased, resulting in both earlier and higher blood alcohol concentration peaks, accompanied by a greater feeling of drunkenness.[55] In addition, there is decreased clearance of alcohol through first-pass mechanism because of decreased availability of alcohol dehydrogenase.[54,56] In practical terms, peak blood alcohol levels achieved after consuming about 2 drinks in women who have had RYGB surgery resemble those observed after consuming about 4 drinks in women who have not had surgery.[55] The data suggest that the legal driving limit in the United States can be exceeded within 10 minutes after drinking.[57]

Alcohol metabolism after SG may also be affected. However, studies have been conflicting, largely because of methodological differences in the measurement of alcohol levels following ingestion (breath vs arterialized blood).[58,59]

Large prospective observational studies show that the prevalence of alcohol use disorder after RYGB increases over time, whereas there seems to be no change in prevalence of alcohol use disorder after adjustable gastric banding.[60,61] Five years after undergoing RYGB, the cumulative incidence of alcohol use disorder symptoms was about 20%.[60] Self-reported problematic alcohol use after RYGB is also higher after RYGB than after laparoscopic adjustable gastric banding.[61] The risk of problematic alcohol use or alcohol use disorder after SG is unknown at this time because of the paucity of good-quality studies.

Assessment of certain risk factors may help identify at-risk patients. Male sex, younger age, smoking, and any alcohol consumption presurgery are associated with increased risk of alcohol use disorder after RYGB.[60–62] Although baseline alcohol consumption is a risk factor, about 20% of patients diagnosed with alcohol use disorder within 5 years of RYGB reported no alcohol consumption in the year before surgery.[61]

In summary, patients undergoing bariatric surgery should be screened for and counseled on the effects of alcohol before and after surgery. Although a history of prior alcohol use disorder is not a contraindication to bariatric surgery, active alcohol use disorder is a contraindication per published guidelines.[63] All patients, regardless of their alcohol use status before surgery, should be made aware that alcohol use disorder can occur in the long term after RYGB in particular.

PREGNANCY AFTER BARIATRIC SURGERY

It is estimated that at least 50% of women who go through bariatric surgery are of childbearing age.[64] It is therefore prudent to include counseling on pregnancy and its outcomes in patients who may become pregnant in the years following bariatric surgery. Although limited, the data generally support improvement in fertility rates following bariatric surgery.[65] In patients with coexisting polycystic ovarian syndrome, bariatric surgery can lead to normalization of menstrual cycles, decreased circulating androgen levels, and improved insulin sensitivity.[66,67]

Bariatric surgery carries with it the risk of nutritional deficiencies, as described in detail previously. Women who have gone through bariatric surgery and who are contemplating pregnancy should be counseled on the appropriate vitamin and mineral supplementation regimen and screened for common nutritional deficiencies before conception. Women who have undergone more malabsorptive procedures, such as the duodenal switch, should be screened for fat-soluble vitamin deficiencies (vitamins A, E), zinc, copper, and other trace elements as dictated by symptoms. Patients with multiple nutritional deficiencies should also be considered for treatment of small intestinal bacterial overgrowth. Current guidelines recommend monitoring for nutritional deficiency every trimester.[63] Pregnant women who have previously undergone adjustable gastric banding should have the band adjusted to allow appropriate weight gain for fetal growth.

Special consideration should be given to screening for gestational diabetes mellitus (GDM) in women who have undergone RYGB. The standard 50-g oral glucose tolerance test (OGTT) is poorly tolerated because it may precipitate dumping and delayed hypoglycemia. Studies have shown serial fasting glucose measurements to have equivalent sensitivity but lower specificity compared with the OGTT.[68] Other alternatives that have been studied include serial monitoring of fasting and 2-hour postprandial glucose and glycated hemoglobin levels.[69,70] At this time, there is no consensus on the optimal screening method for GDM in pregnant women who have previously undergone RYGB.

There have been several retrospective studies and a large case-control cohort investigating pregnancy outcomes in patients who have previously undergone RYGB. The largest study to date, using a Swedish birth register, compared a cohort of pregnant women who had undergone bariatric surgery with those who had not.[71] Ninety-eight percent of the women who had bariatric surgery underwent RYGB, with a mean interval from surgery to conception of 1.1 years. Women who had the RYGB had a lower prevalence of GDM and large-for-gestational-age infants, although there was a slightly higher risk of small-for-gestational-age infants and preterm birth.

Pregnancy outcomes after SG are also favorable based on published retrospective data. In 1 study with mean time from surgery to conception of 1.4 years, a cohort of pregnant women were matched to women of similar preoperative BMI who had not gone through bariatric surgery.[72] There were lower rates of GDM, nonelective caesarean sections, large-for-gestational-age infants, and macrosomia in the group that had undergone surgery. In contrast, there were more infants with low birth weight and small for gestational age in the post-SG group. Mothers in this group also required intravenous iron supplementation more frequently than women in the control group. Similar smaller studies confirm these findings.[73,74] With the laparoscopic SG now being the most commonly performed bariatric procedure in the United States and globally, this information could form an important part of preoperative counseling.

There are additional risks specific to alterations in anatomy, such as the risk of an internal hernia in the Peterson space, which most commonly occurs in the third trimester and is best detected by MRI.[75] Clinical suspicion for this condition should be high in pregnant patients presenting with abdominal pain late in pregnancy.

At present, guidelines recommend that pregnancy is avoided for at least 12 months following bariatric surgery, although the optimal timing of pregnancy following surgery is unknown.[33] There seem to be differences in pregnancy outcomes between the different types of surgery, with at least 1 group reporting that pregnancy within the first year of SG may not be different from pregnancy 1 year after SG.[72] An individualized approach may be suitable, particularly in women who have undergone SG and who do not wish to delay pregnancy, as long as risks and benefits are clearly delineated. However, for all other women, the authors adhere to guideline recommendations that call for a delay in pregnancy following bariatric surgery.

DISCLOSURE

The authors have nothing to disclose.

REFERENCES

1. Buchwald H, Avidor H, Brauwald E, et al. Bariatric surgery: a systematic review and meta-anlysis. JAMA 2004;292:1724–37.
2. Jurgensen JA, Reidt W, Kellogg T, et al. Impact of patient attrition from bariatric surgery practice on clinical outcomes. Obes Surg 2019;29(2):579–84.
3. Roust LR, DiBaise JK. Nutrient deficiencies prior to bariatric surgery. Curr Opin Clin Nutr Metab Care 2017;20(2):138–44.
4. Parrott J, Frank L, Rabena R, et al. American Society for Metabolic and Bariatric Surgery Integrated Health Nutritional Guidelines for the Surgical Weight Loss Patient 2016 Update: micronutrients. Surg Obesity Relat Diseases 2016;13:727–41.
5. Caron M, Hould FS, Lescelleur O, et al. Long-term nutritional impact of sleeve gastrectomy. Surg Obes Relat Dis 2017;13(10):1664–73.
6. Aron-Wisnewsky J, Verger EO, Bounaix C, et al. Nutritional and protein deficiencies in the short term following both gastric bypass and gastric banding. PLoS One 2016;11(2):e0149588.
7. Kumar R, Lieske JC, Collazo-Clavell ML, et al. Fat malabsorption and increased intestinal oxalate absorption are common after Roux-en-Y gastric bypass surgery. Surgery 2011;149(5):654–61.
8. Sanchez A, Rojas P, Basfi-Fer K, et al. Micronutrient deficiencies in morbidly obese women prior to bariatric surgery. Obes Surg 2016;26(2):361–8.
9. Schafer AL, Weaver CM, Black DM, et al. Intestinal calcium absorption decreases dramatically after gastric bypass surgery despite optimization of vitamin D status. J Bone Miner Res 2015;30(8):1377–85.
10. Buchwald H, Oien DM. Metabolic/bariatric surgery worldwide 2011. Obes Surg 2013;23(4):427–36.
11. Strain GW, Torghabeh MH, Gagner M, et al. Nutrient status 9 years after biliopancreatic diversion with duodenal switch (BPD/DS): an observational study. Obes Surg 2017;27(7):1709–18.
12. Topart P, Becouarn G, Delarue J. Weight loss and nutritional outcomes 10 years after biliopancreatic diversion with duodenal switch. Obes Surg 2017;27(7):1645–50.
13. Nett P, Borbely Y, Kroll D. Micronutrient supplementation after biliopancreatic diversion with duodenal switch in the long term. Obes Surg 2016;26(10):2469–74.
14. Lebel S, Dion G, Marceau S, et al. Clinical outcomes of duodenal switch with a 200-cm common channel: a matched, controlled trial. Surg Obes Relat Dis 2016;12(5):1014–20.
15. Papamargaritis D, Aasheim ET, Sampson B, et al. Copper, selenium and zinc levels after bariatric surgery in patients recommended to take multivitamin-mineral supplementation. J Trace Elem Med Biol 2015;31:167–72.
16. James H, Lorentz P, Collazo-Clavell ML. Patient-reported adherence to empiric vitamin/mineral supplementation and related nutrient deficiencies after Roux-en-Y Gastric Bypass. Obes Surg 2016;26(11):2661–6.
17. Peterson LA, Zeng X, Caufield-Noll CP, et al. Vitamin D status and supplementation before and after bariatric surgery: a comprehensive literature review. Surgery for Obesity and Related Diseases 2016;12(3):693–702.
18. Stein EM, Silverberg SJ. Bone loss after bariatric surgery: causes, consequences, and management. Lancet Diabetes Endocrinol 2014;2(2):165–74.
19. Rousseau C, Sean S, Gamache P, et al. Change in fracture risk and fracture pattern after bariatric surgery: nested case-control study. BMJ 2016;354:i3794.

20. Ben-Porat T, Elazary R, Sherf-Dagan S, et al. Bone health following bariatric surgery: implications for management strategies to attenuate bone loss. Adv Nutr 2018;9(2):114–27.
21. Zibellini J, Seimon RV, Lee CM, et al. Does diet-induced weight loss lead to bone loss in overweight or obese adults? A systematic review and meta-analysis of clinical trials. J Bone Miner Res 2015;30(12):2168–78.
22. Shapses SA, Sukumar D. Bone metabolism in obesity and weight loss. Annu Rev Nutr 2012;32:287–309.
23. Gregory NS. The effects of bariatric surgery on bone metabolism. Endocrinol Metab Clin North Am 2017;46(1):105–16.
24. Clarke BL, Khosla S. Female reproductive system and bone. Arch Biochem Biophys 2010;503(1):118–28.
25. Muschitz C, Kocijan R, Haschka J, et al. The impact of Vitamin D, calcium, protein supplementation, and physical exercise on bone metabolism after bariatric surgery: the BABS study. J Bone Miner Res 2016;31(3):672–82.
26. Campanha-Versiani L, Pereira DAG, Ribeiro-Samora GA, et al. The effect of a muscle weight-bearing and aerobic exercise program on the body composition, muscular strength, biochemical markers, and bone mass of obese patients who have undergone gastric bypass surgery. Obes Surg 2017;27(8):2129–37.
27. Semins MJ, Shore AD, Makary MA, et al. The association of increasing body mass index and kidney stone disease. J Urol 2010;183(2):571–5.
28. Lieske JC, Mehta RA, Milliner DS, et al. Kidney stones are common after bariatric surgery. Kidney Int 2015;87(4):839–45.
29. Bhatti UH, Duffy AJ, Roberts KE, et al. Nephrolithiasis after bariatric surgery: a review of pathophysiologic mechanisms and procedural risk. Int J Surg 2016; 36(Pt D):618–23.
30. Park AM, Storm DW, Fulmer BR, et al. A prospective study of risk factors for nephrolithiasis after Roux-en-Y gastric bypass surgery. J Urol 2009;182(5):2334–9.
31. Agrawal V, Liu XJ, Campfield T, et al. Calcium oxalate supersaturation increases early after Roux-en-Y gastric bypass. Surg Obes Relat Dis 2014;10(1):88–94.
32. Sinha MK, Collazo-Clavell ML, Rule A, et al. Hyperoxaluric nephrolithiasis is a complication of Roux-en-Y gastric bypass surgery. Kidney Int 2007;72(1):100–7.
33. Mechanick JI, Apovian C, Brethauer S, et al. Clinical practice guidelines for the perioperative nutritional, metabolic, and nonsurgical support of the bariatric surgery patient–2013 update: cosponsored by American Association of Clinical Endocrinologists, The Obesity Society, and American Society for Metabolic & Bariatric Surgery. Obesity (Silver Spring) 2013;21(Suppl 1):S1–27.
34. Canales BK, Hatch M. Kidney stone incidence and metabolic urinary changes after modern bariatric surgery: review of clinical studies, experimental models, and prevention strategies. Surg Obes Relat Dis 2014;10(4):734–42.
35. Service GJ, Thompson GB, Service FJ, et al. Hyperinsulinemic hypoglycemia with nesidioblastosis after gastric-bypass surgery. N Engl J Med 2005;353(3): 249–54.
36. Salehi M, Vella A, McLaughlin T, et al. Hypoglycemia after gastric bypass surgery: current concepts and controversies. J Clin Endocrinol Metab 2018; 103(8):2815–26.
37. Goldfine AB, Patti ME. How common is hypoglycemia after gastric bypass? Obesity (Silver Spring) 2016;24(6):1210–1.
38. Marsk R, Jonas E, Rasmussen F, et al. Nationwide cohort study of post-gastric bypass hypoglycaemia including 5,040 patients undergoing surgery for obesity in 1986-2006 in Sweden. Diabetologia 2010;53(11):2307–11.

39. Kefurt R, Langer FB, Schindler K, et al. Hypoglycemia after Roux-En-Y gastric bypass: detection rates of continuous glucose monitoring (CGM) versus mixed meal test. Surgery for Obesity and Related Diseases 2015;11(3):564–9.
40. Salehi M, Gastaldelli A, D'Alessio DA. Altered islet function and insulin clearance cause hyperinsulinemia in gastric bypass patients with symptoms of postprandial hypoglycemia. Journal of Clinical Endocrinology & Metabolism 2014;99(6): 2008–17.
41. Shah M, Law JH, Micheletto F, et al. Contribution of endogenous glucagon-like peptide 1 to glucose metabolism after Roux-en-Y gastric bypass. Diabetes 2014;63(2):483–93.
42. Tack J, Arts J, Caenepeel P, et al. Pathophysiology, diagnosis and management of postoperative dumping syndrome. Nat Rev Gastroenterol Hepatol 2009;6(10): 583–90.
43. Goldfine AB, Mun EC, Devine E, et al. Patients with neuroglycopenia after gastric bypass surgery have exaggerated incretin and insulin secretory responses to a mixed meal. J Clin Endocrinol Metab 2007;92(12):4678–85.
44. Laferrere B, Teixeira J, McGinty J, et al. Effect of weight loss by gastric bypass surgery versus hypocaloric diet on glucose and incretin levels in patients with type 2 diabetes. J Clin Endocrinol Metab 2008;93(7):2479–85.
45. Salehi M, Gastaldelli A, D'Alessio DA. Blockade of glucagon-like peptide 1 receptor corrects postprandial hypoglycemia after gastric bypass. Gastroenterology 2014;146(3):669–80.e2.
46. Honka H, Salehi M. Postprandial hypoglycemia after gastric bypass surgery: from pathogenesis to diagnosis and treatment. Curr Opin Clin Nutr Metab Care 2019; 22(4):295–302.
47. Suhl E, Anderson-Haynes SE, Mulla C, et al. Medical nutrition therapy for post-bariatric hypoglycemia: practical insights. Surg Obes Relat Dis 2017;13(5): 888–96.
48. Myint KS, Greenfield JR, Farooqi IS, et al. Prolonged successful therapy for hyperinsulinaemic hypoglycaemia after gastric bypass: the pathophysiological role of GLP1 and its response to a somatostatin analogue. Eur J Endocrinol 2012;166(5):951–5.
49. Abrahamsson N, Engström BE, Sundbom M, et al. GLP1 analogs as treatment of postprandial hypoglycemia following gastric bypass surgery: a potential new indication? Eur J Endocrinol 2013;169(6):885–9.
50. Stier C, Chiappetta S. Endoluminal Revision (OverStitch (TM) , Apollo Endosurgery) of the Dilated Gastroenterostomy in Patients with Late Dumping Syndrome After Proximal Roux-en-Y Gastric Bypass. Obes Surg 2016;26(8):1978–84.
51. Davis DB, Khoraki J, Ziemelis M, et al. Roux en Y gastric bypass hypoglycemia resolves with gastric feeding or reversal: confirming a non-pancreatic etiology. Mol Metab 2018;9:15–27.
52. Vanderveen KA, Grant CS, Thompson GB, et al. Outcomes and quality of life after partial pancreatectomy for noninsulinoma pancreatogenous hypoglycemia from diffuse islet cell disease. Surgery 2010;148(6):1237–45 [discussion: 1245–6].
53. Klockhoff H, Naslund I, Jones AW. Faster absorption of ethanol and higher peak concentration in women after gastric bypass surgery. Br J Clin Pharmacol 2002; 54(6):587–91.
54. Hagedorn JC, Encarnacion B, Brat GA, et al. Does gastric bypass alter alcohol metabolism? Surg Obes Relat Dis 2007;3(5):543–8 [discussion: 548].
55. Pepino MY, Okunade AL, Eagon J C, et al. Effect of Roux-en-Y Gastric Bypass Surgery: Converting 2 Alcoholic Drinks to 4. JAMA Surg 2015;150(11):1096–8.

56. Gentry RT, Baraona E, Lieber CS. Agonist: gastric first pass metabolism of alcohol. J Lab Clin Med 1994;123(1):21–6 [discussion: 27].
57. Steffen KJ, Engel SG, Pollert GA, et al. Blood alcohol concentrations rise rapidly and dramatically after Roux-en-Y gastric bypass. Surg Obes Relat Dis 2013;9(3):470–3.
58. Acevedo MB, Ferrando R, Patterson BW, et al. Effect of alcohol ingestion on plasma glucose kinetics after Roux-en-Y gastric bypass surgery. Surg Obes Relat Dis 2019;15(1):36–42.
59. Gallo AS, Berducci MA, Nijhawan S, et al. Alcohol metabolism is not affected by sleeve gastrectomy. Surg Endosc 2015;29(5):1088–93.
60. King WC, Chen JY, Courcoulas AP, et al. Alcohol and other substance use after bariatric surgery: prospective evidence from a U.S. multicenter cohort study. Surg Obes Relat Dis 2017;13(8):1392–402.
61. Svensson PA, Anveden Å, Romeo S, et al. Alcohol consumption and alcohol problems after bariatric surgery in the Swedish obese subjects study. Obesity (Silver Spring) 2013;21(12):2444–51.
62. King WC, Chen JY, Mitchell JE, et al. Prevalence of alcohol use disorders before and after bariatric surgery. JAMA 2012;307(23):2516–25.
63. Mechanick JI, Youdim A, Jones DB, et al. Clinical practice guidelines for the perioperative nutritional, metabolic, and nonsurgical support of the bariatric surgery patient–2013 update: cosponsored by American Association of Clinical Endocrinologists, the Obesity Society, and American Society for Metabolic & Bariatric Surgery. Endocr Pract 2013;19(2):337–72.
64. Maggard MA, Yermilov I, Li Z, et al. Pregnancy and fertility following bariatric surgery: a systematic review. JAMA 2008;300(19):2286–96.
65. Musella M, Milone M, Bellini M, et al. Effect of bariatric surgery on obesity-related infertility. Surg Obes Relat Dis 2012;8(4):445–9.
66. Escobar-Morreale HF, Botella-Carretero JI, Alvarez-Blasco F, et al. The polycystic ovary syndrome associated with morbid obesity may resolve after weight loss induced by bariatric surgery. J Clin Endocrinol Metab 2005;90(12):6364–9.
67. Teitelman M, Grotegut CA, Williams NN, et al. The impact of bariatric surgery on menstrual patterns. Obes Surg 2006;16(11):1457–63.
68. Donovan L, Hartling L, Muise M, et al. Screening tests for gestational diabetes: a systematic review for the U.S. Preventive Services Task Force. Ann Intern Med 2013;159(2):115–22.
69. American College of Obstetricians and Gynecologists. ACOG practice bulletin no. 105: bariatric surgery and pregnancy. Obstet Gynecol 2009;113(6):1405–13.
70. Rajput R, Yogesh Yadav, Rajput M, et al. Utility of HbA1c for diagnosis of gestational diabetes mellitus. Diabetes Res Clin Pract 2012;98(1):104–7.
71. Johansson K, Stephansson O, Neovius M. Outcomes of pregnancy after bariatric surgery. N Engl J Med 2015;372(23):2267.
72. Rottenstreich A, Levin G, Kleinstern G, et al. The effect of surgery-to-conception interval on pregnancy outcomes after sleeve gastrectomy. Surg Obes Relat Dis 2018;14(12):1795–803.
73. Basbug A, Ellibeş Kaya A, Dogan S, et al. Does pregnancy interval after laparoscopic sleeve gastrectomy affect maternal and perinatal outcomes? J Matern Fetal Neonatal Med 2019;32(22):3764–70.
74. Han SM, Kim WW, Moon R, et al. Pregnancy outcomes after laparoscopic sleeve gastrectomy in morbidly obese Korean patients. Obes Surg 2013;23(6):756–9.
75. Vannevel V, Jans G, Bialecka M, et al. Internal herniation in pregnancy after gastric bypass: a systematic review. Obstet Gynecol 2016;127(6):1013–20.

76. Cadegiani FA, Silva OS. Acarbose promotes remission of both early and late dumping syndromes in post-bariatric patients. Diabetes Metab Syndr Obes 2016;9:443–6.
77. Spanakis E, Gragnoli C. Successful medical management of status post-Roux-en-Y-gastric-bypass hyperinsulinemic hypoglycemia. Obes Surg 2009;19(9): 1333–4.
78. Gonzalez-Gonzalez A, Delgado M, Fraga-Fuentes MD. Use of diazoxide in management of severe postprandial hypoglycemia in patient after Roux-en-Y gastric bypass. Surg Obes Relat Dis 2013;9(1):e18–9.

Printed and bound by CPI Group (UK) Ltd, Croydon, CR0 4YY

08/05/2025

01864691-0008